Tales of the Exam Room Volume 4: **Scary Medical Stories**

This is a work of fiction. Unless otherwise stated – all names, characters, businesses, places, events, locales, and incidents in this book are the product of either the author's imagination or are used in a fictitious manner. Any resemblance to actual persons, living or dead, or actual events is purely coincidental.

ISBN: 978-1-954814-05-9 (Paperback)

ISBN: 978-1-954814-04-2 (EBook)

First Edition 2021.

Credits:

Book Cover and Formatting by: farhanshahid101

Obsidian Wolf Publishing

PO Box 1086 Salem, UT 84653

Contents

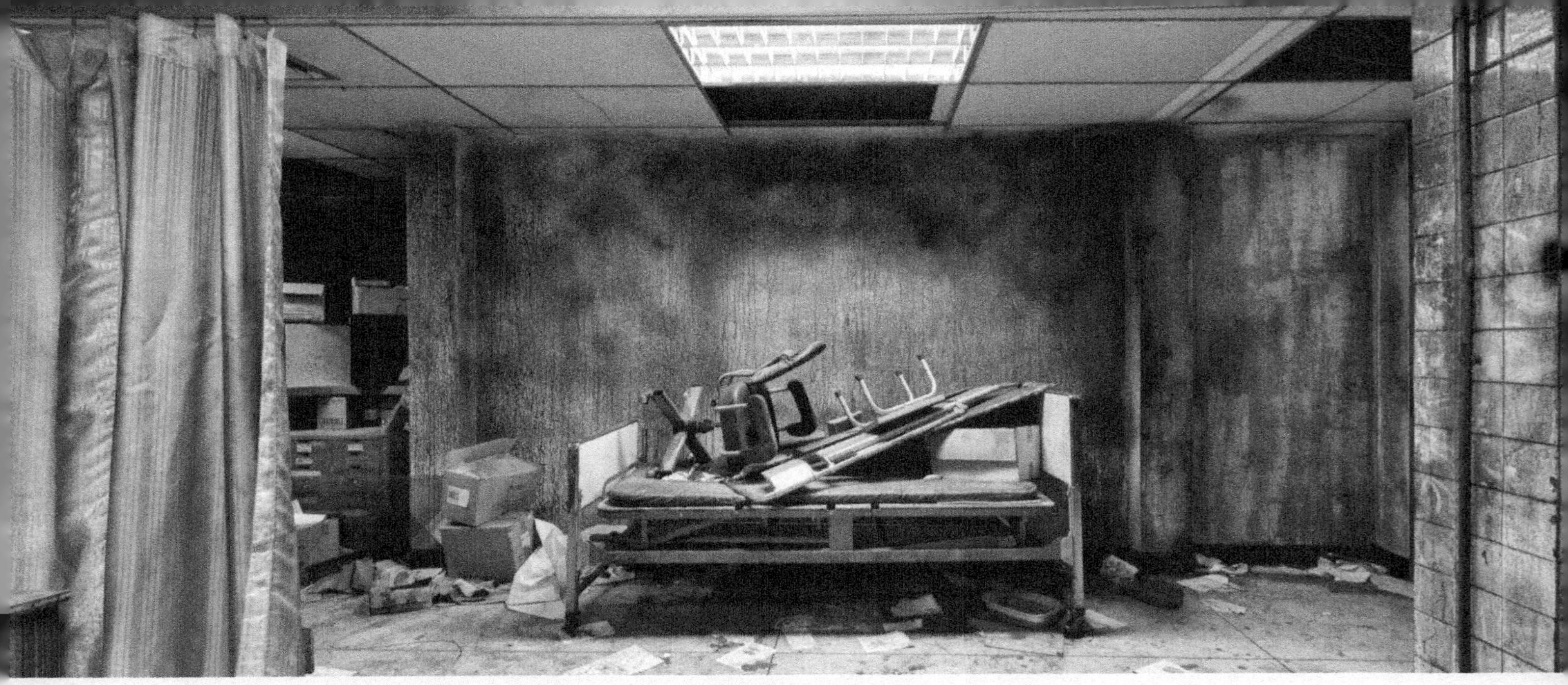

Introduction

Scary Medical Stories: Tales of the Exam Room – Vol 4.

The stories of medicine should be told, felt, discussed, and retold over and over again. There is so much to learn about patient encounters, decision-making disasters, and incredible actions of those involved during odd and life-saving situations. Whether you come to this book hoping to learn more about medicine or searching for the crazy and unexpected stories that are taking place all around you. You have come to the right place. This is our 4th volume of short stories, and the other volumes are just as exciting.

We have collected scary medical stories from a variety of different places and medical circumstances. We have changed the names, locations, and often the situations to protect privacy and to provide a slightly more entertainment value.

This book is intended to cause the reader to shake their heads or question whether a particular episode truly happened. Most people love sitting around the dinner table or a campfire listening to unforeseen stories.

Volume 4 takes a look at some of the extreme sides of medicine, including a boy who gets hit in the chest with a baseball and an unrelenting episode of vomiting, and more. These stories may give you a few chills, so be prepared.

Remember that the art of medicine is seldom straightforward. There are many boring cases of sore throat and back pain, but we want to shine on the erratic and unstable behavior cases.

Please Enjoy and Feel free to Join Us for additional medical stories at examroomtales.com

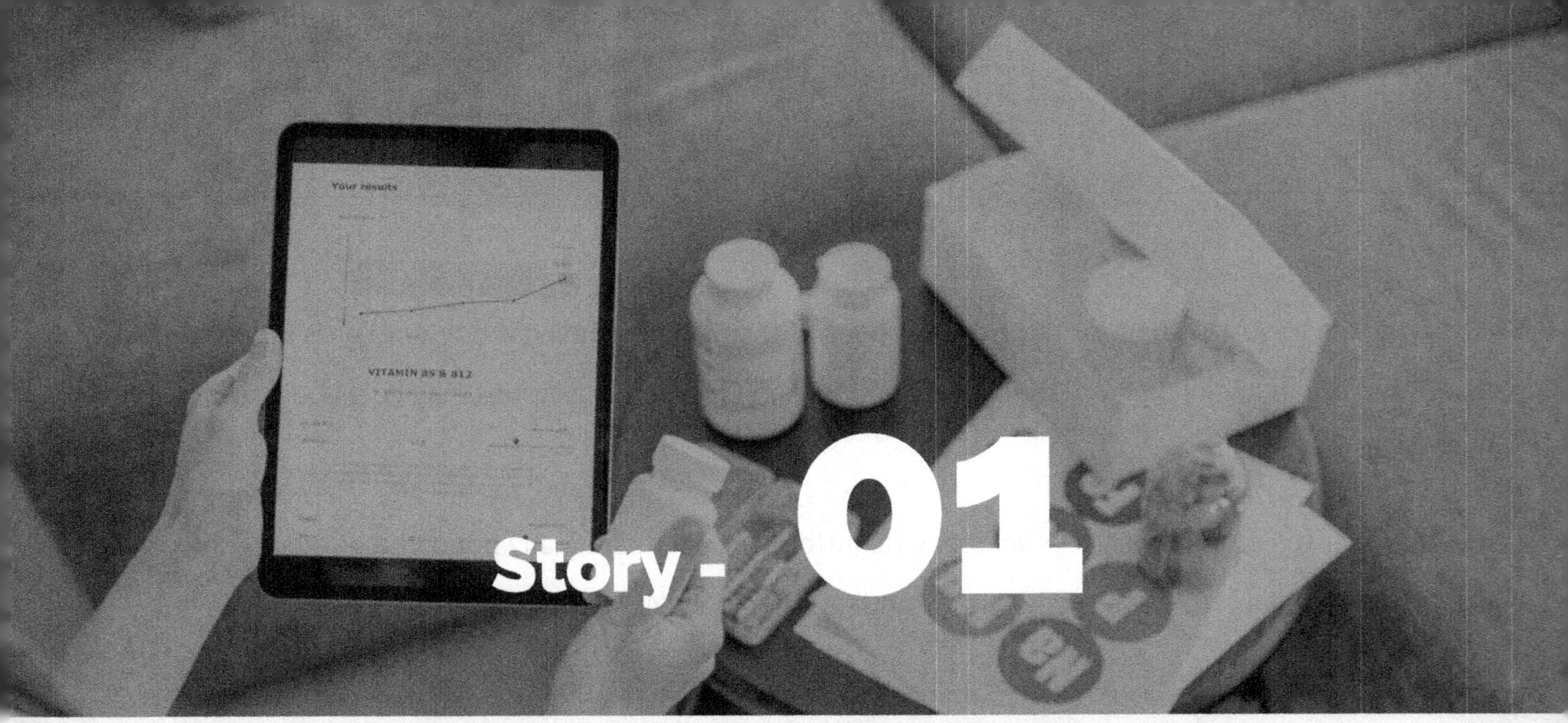

Story - 01

Book Slamming a Bible Cyst

I can't tell you how often I see patients and the first thing out of their mouth is . . . ***"I read on the internet."***

Now don't get me wrong, there is a lot of information on the internet and some of it is good and some . . . not so good. But trust me, if you want life-saving information and treatment on cancer diagnosis, post-menopausal bleeding, heart attacks, medication side effects, and many more - Go to the professionals!!!

Robert was my patient for the day - and he has been good-natured enough to let me share this story.

When I entered the exam room - Robert had a large glove on his right hand. When he took it off, there was some redness, bruising, swelling, and a whole lot more.

Treatment Regimen

Robert explained that he started having these nodules on his right hand and they were painful, swollen, and red a few weeks before. Like many people, going to the doctor was the last thing he wanted. He thought about his "injury" for a day or so and thought that he might have hit his hand at work. He knew that NSAIDs help with swelling so he started taking IBU three times a day for several days. He felt some relief and thought that he had solved the problem. Despite the pain improvement, he started noticing more and more areas of swelling.

He finally admitted to himself that he hadn't injured his hand at work and so he wondered if the swelling could be caused by inflammation. He thought that this was a logical idea. So, for the next 24 hours, he was putting an ice pack on his hand every twenty minutes and resting for an hour or so.

His hand became super cold - but no improvement. He tried some creams, Tylenol, and finally a heating pad to improve circulation.

Research on the Internet

Robert sat down at his computer and began searching the internet about hand redness. There were several things that popped up - Infection, Inflammation, Spider bites, and STDs.

Robert admits that at this moment, he started freaking out. He was glad to see that he hadn't been too far off the mark with Inflammation. The rest of the things sounded pretty bad. To him, the most likely culprit was an infection. For the next two nights - he took as much triple antibiotic cream and lathered his hand. Nothing helped, in fact, it was now starting to look like he had some boils under his asking and thought that they were pus pockets. In the clinic, he admitted that he took a needle and tried to pop one of the areas on his knuckles. He wasn't able to get out of any infection.

Having a Frank Discussion with his Wife

For Robert, this part was the most embarrassing. He read that some STDs - such as Gonorrhea can cause Gonococcal arthritis in joints. It affects women more often but Robert had the brilliant idea to bring it up at dinner. His wife had been asking him for the past several days to go see his doctor. He'd refused but he decided a mealtime discussion about sexual partners was a good idea. He slept on the couch that evening. This was the day before he came into the doctor's clinic needing more treatment.

Back to the Internet

Later that night, he began looking into cysts of the hands, on the internet. The first thing he clicked on was Ganglion cyst. He read that these are non-cancerous cysts that commonly develop on the tendons of the wrists and the joints of the hands. Sometimes they go away on their own, sometimes they need to be drained or surgery, and sometimes there is a more alternative treatment.

He read that these cysts have been around for a long time - meaning that they were seen many years ago. Treatment would consist of hitting the cysts with a bible or the largest book around. This is probably more of an urban legend and NOT the recommended treatment. However, Robert was desperate. He found his bible and began hitting his hands. Needless to say, nothing happened but some more swelling, pain, and bruising.

The Actual Diagnosis

Inside my clinic, Robert and I were able to discuss the cause for his bumps and lumps and even the appearance of a boil-like infection on his hand. He had been suffering from joint pains, fever, and chills for a few weeks by now and nothing had helped.

The actual diagnosis is something called Tophi Gout. And you guessed it - the root cause is gout. Gout often causes problems in the joints. We did a blood test and began the correct treatment immediately. In a matter of days, he noticed an improvement. He was having a flare-up and receiving the right treatment was largely beneficial.

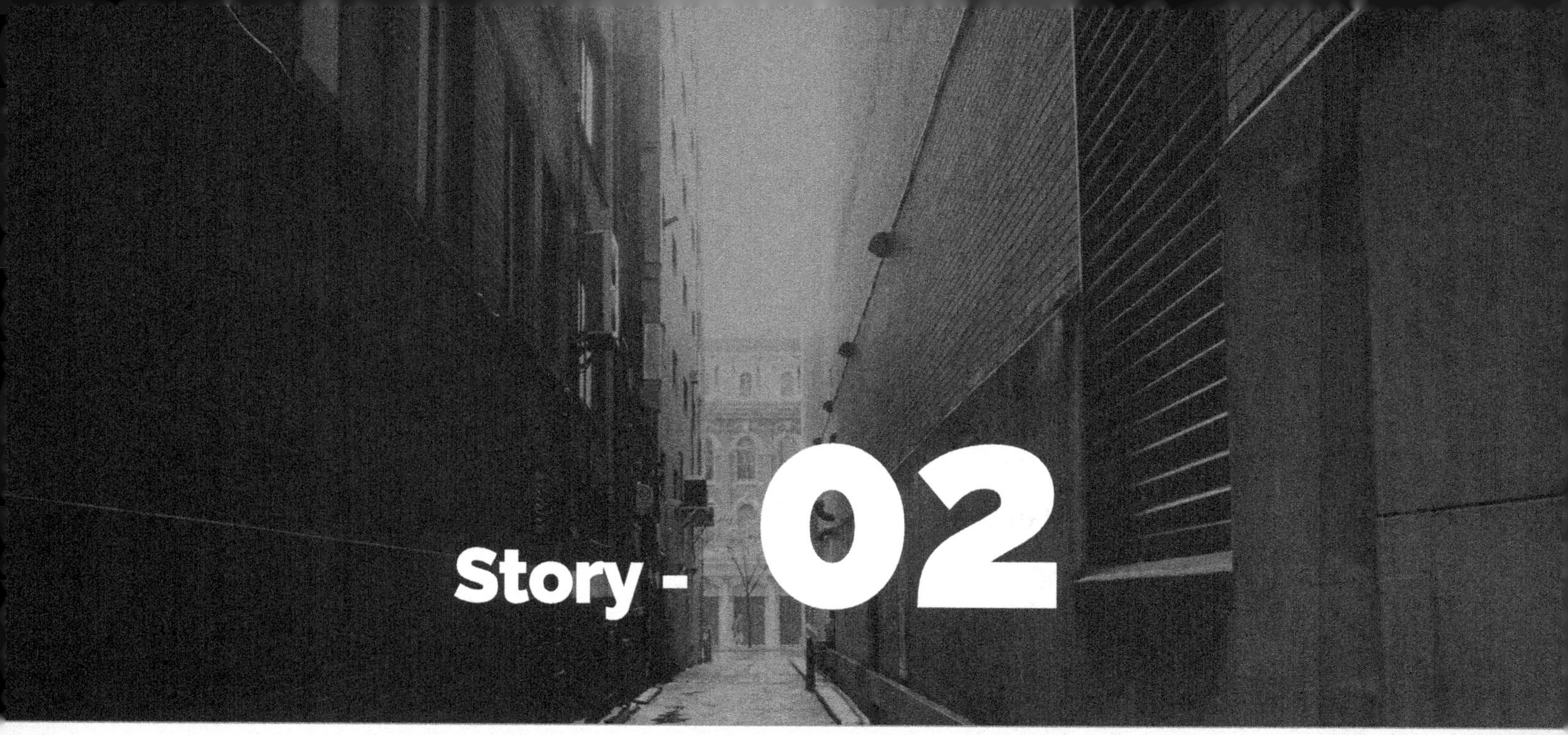

Substantial Injury Following a Fall in an Alley

Pain can make all rational thoughts disappear, and you may begin acting on instinct. Imagine having the worst pain imaginable and knowing that someone else had caused that pain intentionally.

Blake Buckley was found in an alley with significant trauma to his head. There was a large pool of blood, and Blake was barely conscious. He was wearing black jeans and a black hoodie. It was nearly two in the morning. Blake's screams brought several people running into the alley to find him suffering from a significant medical injury. An ambulance was called for immediately by some of the bystanders.

Upon arrival, the paramedics instantly recognized this situation as potentially life-threatening and one of the strangest they had ever encountered. The patient was still breathing, which was incredibly important. The wound was primarily around the facial features. The neck, lungs, and lower portion of the body were without injury; at least none that they could see. They insisted on being cautious as they proceeded in stabilizing their patient.

The first paramedic brought over the gurney and a backboard. Blake was positioned onto his back on top of the gurney. Spider straps were used to bind Blake to the backboard, and a plastic neck brace was attached, preventing Blake from moving his head back and forth. With the help of another two paramedics, he was lifted onto the gurney and transported to the ambulance. Blake's vitals were stable, and he was breathing steadily. But that could change at any time.

Blake only asked one question, "Is my face going to be alright?"

No one answered.

Inside the ambulance, an IV was started, and they began to wrap a dressing around the head wound. They were unable to place a nasal canula for oxygen, but fortunately, Blake's O2 sats (oxygen saturation) remained normal. The drive to the hospital took 10 minutes. Halfway there, the pain kicked in and Blake began moaning, and his hands opened and closed repeatedly. There was palpable concern that Blake would take a turn for the worse.

The paramedics removed Blake from the ambulance and transferred care to the Emergency Room nurses. An explanation of the patient's situation and vitals were given to the charge nurse as Blake was wheeled into an exam room.

The nurses began to do a new set of vitals and to ensure the patient was still stable. The doctor arrived a few minutes later, and an X-ray was immediately ordered. Less than five minutes later, they took Blake for a facial X-ray along with the neck and his entire back. When he came back into his room, the doctor was waiting to hear the story of what had happened.

Doctor Flanders asked, "Mr. Buckley, can you tell us what happened?"

Blake was still lying on the backboard, and it was difficult for him to speak. He managed to say, "I went to Club V earlier tonight. As I was leaving, I was walking to my car. I had to park on Ocean Avenue, it was the only spot I could find."

"Continue."

"I left the club after one in the morning." Blake took a moment to gather his energy. He continued, "I was a block away from my car when someone jumped out of the shadows and demanded my money. I took off running and somehow got all mixed up. I must've run into this alley to hide. I remember tripping over something, and my head smacked into something. It hurt so bad. I can't believe that I have a women's heel sticking in my face. What is going to happen with my eye?"

"I am waiting for the X-ray results so I can see if there is any more damage. We also need to know if we can take you off this backboard and remove the C-collar. I don't know if we are going to be able to save the eye and if we do, we are extremely worried about your vision and possible infection. You have the stiletto heel embedded in your eye. I am shocked that you are still conscious. We'll need to take you in for surgery and remove it, but that is down the line an hour or so."

"What are we waiting for?" demanded Blake.

"X-ray clearance and to hear your side of the story. As I said before, there could be additional damage. We don't want to go into surgery blind. In a few minutes we will get you prepped for surgery."

The surgery lasted for a few hours to remove the three-inch stiletto from the left eye of Blake. In the end, the left eye needed to be completely removed. An orbital implant surgery also occurred. It would take weeks to heal. He was lucky that the stiletto didn't go deeper into the head, possibly injuring the brain. The eye socket was broken, and a plate was required to stabilize the eye. The goal was that at some point in the future, he would be able to use a prosthetic implant.

Hours later, Blake came out of surgery. The nurses asked how he was feeling. He was groggy for another hour or so. He was given some additional medications and slept on and off. By the time he became aware of the people around him, it was late in the afternoon of the next day. To his shock, he had handcuffs on both arms.

After he was taken out of recovery, nurses came in and out of Blake's room, ensuring that his needs were met. He kept asking them questions, but they refused to answer them. A few hours later, a new doctor and a police officer came into Blake's room. Blake protested about having the cuffs on his wrist.

The officer spoke, "Don't worry, Mr. Buckley, everything is going to be fine. However, the story that you gave Dr. Flanders isn't quite how things went. We talked with him after your surgery was finished."

"What are you talking about?" exploded Blake. "Someone tried to mug me."

"Not true," the officer said. "You see, we have a witness with a matching shoe. Her missing shoe matches the one the doctor removed from your eye."

"I don't know what you are talking about. She must have lost her shoe."

"She says that you attacked her and knocked her down. While on the ground and trying to protect herself, she hit you with the shoe and ran away."

"No way," Blake said. "That must've been someone else."

The officer sat on the end of the bed and said, "The funny thing about the alley you were in, they actually have a camera that shows you trying to accost the real victim. You attacked and punched her and tried to force yourself onto her. In self-defense, she got you good. Couldn't be happier myself. You are under arrest."

Blake Buckley spent the next few weeks in the hospital with an officer present the entire time. He was later transferred to jail and subsequently to prison to serve several years for attempted rape.

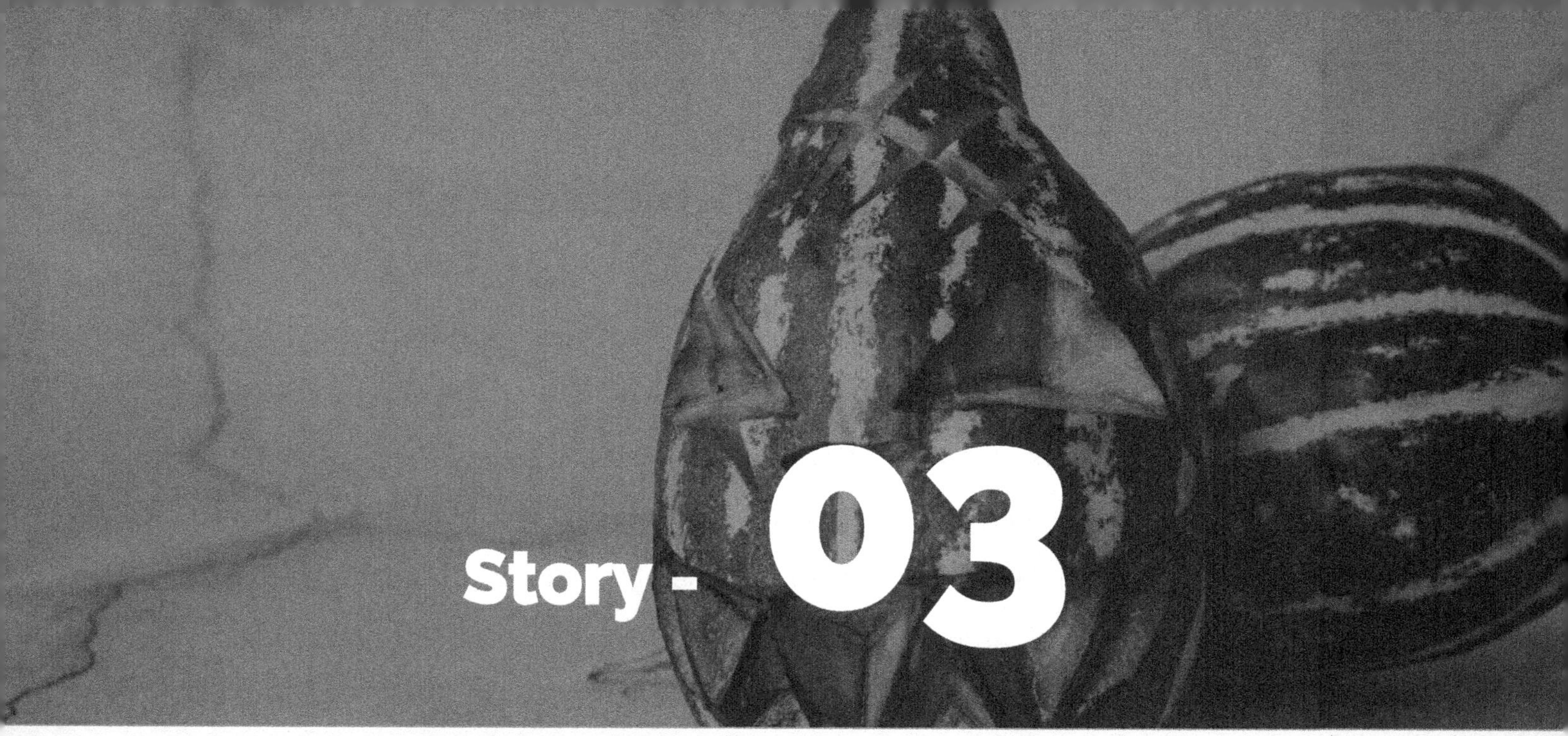

The Green Machine

If you combine Halloween and a full moon, you really have no idea what to expect in the Emergency Room. It was my last shift of four twelve-hour shifts in a row when things began to crash down around us, and I mean literally. The story of the Green Machine is legendary.

Around eleven o'clock, a group of teenagers from a party arrived. They had been playing games and having fun at one of their friends' houses. It had been well chaperoned. Near the end of the night, they started bobbing for apples, eating doughnuts, and drinking punch. Someone had dared the kids to drink as much punch as possible. It seemed like a fun and innocent game. Unbeknown to the group, someone must've spiked their punch because the parents noticed that they were acting pretty crazy. By the time they arrived at the hospital, they were pretty sick. There were five or six kids, and they started vomiting everywhere. It took several nurses to start IVs, give meds, and clean up a large amount of puke.

The next patient to arrive came in from a hit-and-run pedestrian accident. It was a preteen kid who had been out with his friends and was hit by a car that came out of nowhere. The kid had been in costume as a ninja and most of his costume was dark. The car crossed the center line and swiped the kid from the side. None of his friends had even seen the car coming and luckily, they were several steps back when it happened. The car hit the light pole after hitting the kid and drove off. Fortunately, it had only been his leg that had been hit. After a work-up and an X-ray, our staff found that he had a broken leg. The scariest part, it could've been a lot worse.

Thirty minutes later was when my patient arrived. He had been found alone in his room and he was unconscious. At first, his parents thought he wasn't breathing. They called an ambulance, and he was transported to the hospital. On the way over, the kid woke up a few times, but the only thing he said, sounded like gibberish. As he was rushed into the exam room, I noticed that he appeared to be unconscious and asleep. An IV had been placed, and he had been placed on oxygen. The patient was as relaxed as anyone I had ever seen. He was dressed in a scarecrow outfit, clearly from Halloween, but his face was a dark green as if he had paint or makeup applied.

The patient was mostly stable but unable to respond to the doctor trying to start an initial exam. The doctor pulled back his eyelids, checked his vitals, and listened to his heart. The patient was so calm; he didn't seem to have a worry in the world.

"Is this green paint on his face?" asked Dr. Nielson. "Can someone try to wash that off?"

RN Rebecca and I were in the room attending to different things. I began cutting off the costume of the patient. Rebecca said, "I think it might be paint on his face. Does anyone know if he was huffing paint?"

"Go ask the parents," Dr. Nielson asked. "It could also be part of his costume."

Rebecca ran from the room.

That was when the patient's eyes flipped open, and he began fighting Dr. Nielson and me. He grabbed my wrist and started screaming. He said something about apples, sleeping, zombies, and creatures of the dark. His spittle was spraying the room as if he was drooling. He was so strong.

Dr. Nielson said, "Nancy. Grab his wrist. It'll be easier to control the arm."

I followed his advice, and soon we had control of the patient. His eyes were unfocused, and he was staring off at the ceiling. No matter what I said, he could not refocus.

His green face was about as weird as anything I'd ever seen.

The patient said, "Take off my clothes. It is so hot in here."

"I don't think that is paint," Dr. Nielson said. "Something else is going on here."

Rebecca raced back into the room. She said, "The parents are calling their daughter, still at the house. She's going to check his room. This kid's name is Stewart."

"We can't wait. Let's get a tube down to his stomach and give him some charcoal."

"Do you think this an overdose?"

"I'm not sure. This is the best treatment."

It took another nurse and MA to hold Stewart while they put a tube down into his stomach and gave him a large amount of charcoal. The tube went through his nose to make it easier. The goal was for it to bind with anything he might have in his stomach, especially if he overdosed."

Rebecca asked, "Will Charcoal help if he huffed paint?"

"No, it won't. Let's give some meds that might help."

We quickly increased the IV fluids and gave some medications that could help with some of the adverse effects of the symptoms of huffing. Not long afterward, the patient became calmer, but he certainly didn't like anything in his nose and kept trying to pull out the tube. He was still confused, and his eyes fluttered.

"Go check in with the parents again," said Dr. Nielson.

Rebecca left, and most of the charcoal had been administered. The moment Rebecca stepped from the room, Stewart knocked me sideways and stood to leave. His eyes flashed open, and he ran for the door. His IV site was pulled from his arm, and he made it a few steps outside the door before colliding with one of our housekeepers. Both were sent sprawling to the ground. Stewart was captured and taken back into the exam room. More staff came inside and helped hold down the patient to have a second IV and nasogastric placed.

Rebecca returned; she was out of breath. She said, "Sister didn't find any paint cans, but there was a ton of wrappers of Benadryl. Looks like the kid crushed and snorted them."

Dr. Nielson thought about it for a second. He said, "That's why his face is green. It isn't paint but an anticholinergic event. Let's sedate him and put him on a ventilator. Give more charcoal and fluids."

The next few days were rough for Stewart. He had some cardiac changes and abnormal findings in his blood work. But he pulled out of everything alright. He had a lot of explaining to do, especially to his parents. When the day finally came for Stewart to be released from the hospital, he finally told everyone what happened. He didn't remember everything, but his story was unbelievable.

Stewart said, "I have a drug problem and need help. I understand that. I don't remember everything, but I was at this party with some friends, and I thought it would be a good idea to spike the punch. I almost got caught by his mom, and I ran from the house. I was driving home when I hit a light pole. I was pretty spooked, and so when I finally got home, I just wanted to get some sleep. I just wanted the day to be over. I heard that Benadryl helps you sleep, and so I decided to snort some Benadryl. I guess the rest is history."

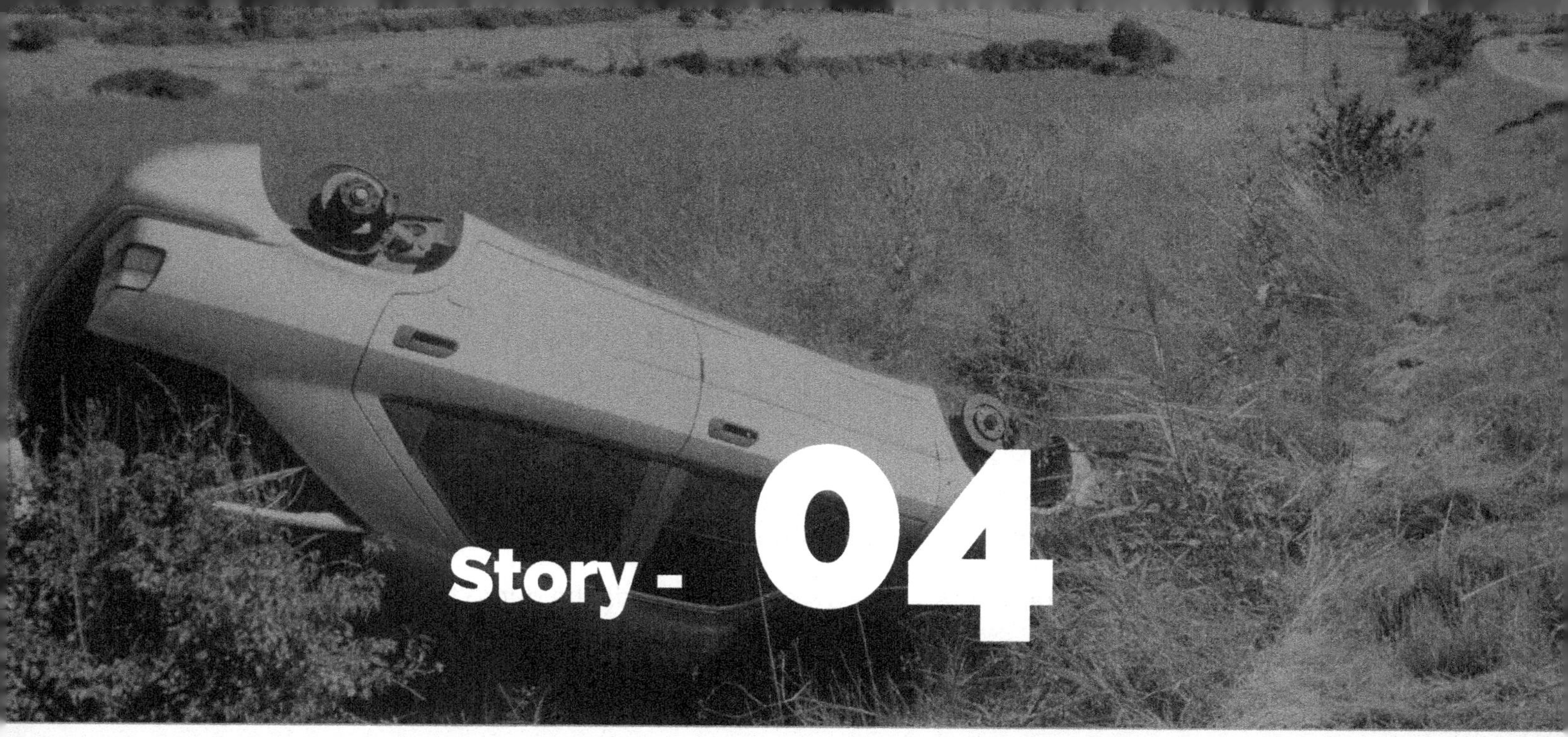

Surprising Car Accident on a Dirt Road

Paramedics arrived at a dirt road completely surprised at what they found. It had been just over thirty minutes from the first phone call to dispatch. Best case scenario, the accident had happened ten or fifteen minutes before that. They weren't sure what they were going to find.

The accident had been unwitnessed, so time was extremely important. The driver who first arrived at the scene thought it couldn't have been more than ten minutes after the original accident. The dirt road went up a slight incline before it swerved to the right. Police reports indicated that a teenager had recently stolen a dump truck from a worksite, and it was believed to be the exact vehicle involved in the crash.

Mr. Morgan had been the first driver on scene. When he stopped and got out of his car, he circled the dump truck, searching for occupants, anyone injured, or any sounds. There were none. He had a pretty good view into the cab, through the window, and found that the front seats were empty. The front glass was cracked and splintered. He next searched the embankment next to the vehicle, and again, found no one. Walking up and down the hill, he shouted for anyone to respond, but the entire area was quiet. In the end, Mr. Morgan felt that whoever was involved in this accident was hiding or had run away. Because he didn't have cell service, in this area, on this road, he hopped back into his car and drove a few miles back down the road to place the call. He had explained all of this to dispatch.

The ambulance arrived as quickly as possible. A firetruck and two police cars arrived mere minutes after the ambulance. Garcia, one of the paramedics, started walking towards the dump truck. The vehicle was on its left side, the same side as a driver would be. He reacted very similarly to Mr. Morgan. After checking the front window, the area around the vehicle, and more—he concluded the same results as Mr. Morgan. However, his training and experience told him that whoever was in this crash had walked away with a pretty severe injury, and he was likely bleeding somewhere in the woods surrounding the road. Soon the newly arrived officers began searching the area for any footprints or other signs of injury.

A tow truck had already been called, and the road had been blocked. The officers and firefighters who had joined the search, found nothing.

Officer Samansky, standing near the truck, yelled, "I hear something. It sounds like gasps." She was bending down near the roof of the vehicle.

The paramedics and an officer sprinted in her direction.

Her senior officer, Officer Blanding, asked, "Are you sure that you heard something from the vehicle?"

"Someone is inside. Listen."

The next sounds were not hard to imagine. The individual trapped somewhere inside had evidently woken up and was screaming. The sounds were unnerving.

"What are our options?" Firefighter Jenkins asked.

Paramedic Garcia said, "See if you can climb onto the vehicle and go in through the passenger door. See what you can see." Garcia moved to the front window and struggled to visualize anyone inside. That's when he saw the arm for the first time. It was caught outside the window somehow. The rest of the body had been pinned above the seat, which was now on its side. The occupant was struggling with the ability to move, but he was clearly in some obvious pain. "I see someone," Garcia shouted. "His arm looks pinned under the vehicle.

The staff worked furiously for the next several minutes. Firefighter Jenkins was inside the vehicle, trying to stabilize the driver. He was in a world of hurt. The first thing Jenkins noticed was that the truck had landed on its side, on an embankment, but that the ground was not smooth. The window appeared to have been rolled down. He could stand on the ground and witnessed that the man's arm was bent unnaturally like it had been sucked underneath the truck. They handed him a shovel, and he began digging at the ground through the side window.

Garcia climbed into the cab found the man in rough shape. He was in significant pain, but his injuries did not appear life threatening. However, the longer the man spent trapped, the less likely he would escape without a bad outcome. The man's head was bleeding, and he had a large gash.

Garcia asked, "What's your name?"

"Hector Brosnan."

"How old are you"?

Garcia learned that the fifty-six-year-old man worked as a dump truck operator. He had been driving and hit some loose gravel when the truck slid and flipped onto his side. The man was twisted and was essentially pinned, because of his arm, to the back window, above the seat. He was in serious pain.

Ten minutes later the dirt around Hector's arm gave way, and his arm could be maneuvered in such a way that he slid down onto the seat. Hector was in bad shape and had worsened over the last few minutes. He was breathing hard, and he was barely conscious at this point. The pain and the situation had been hard to handle. His arm was most likely broken in a few different places, and much of the skin had been torn from the arm. There was blood and damage to almost the entire arm. It appeared as if the arm had been out the window the entire time the truck slid on the ground. Road burn was an understatement.

Jenkins and Garcia maneuvered and finally lifted Hector out of the cab through the passenger window. Furtado, a new paramedic, was ready with the gurney. She and officers Samansky and Blanding helped lift and transport Hector to the gurney. The paramedics began working promptly. They put an air cast around the arm, started an IV in the opposite arm, and strapped the patient to the gurney. He was loaded into the ambulance and was driven to the hospital.

Upon arrival at the hospital, there was a helicopter standing by, and he was transported to a larger hospital closer to the city. The doctor was shocked that Hector had survived such an accident. They had a surgical center ready for him. They had to pick out most of the gravel embedded in his arm, clean the wound before they were able to open the skin and place rods, and fix the fractures in the arms.

Hector suffered a shoulder dislocation, along with a broken arm, a concussion, and some fractured ribs. He was treated at the hospital for several days before being discharged. He required some skin grafts, and other treatments to save the arm.

Hector reported that he was driving his truck on the dirt road with his elbow hanging out of the open window. The truck tipped so fast that he didn't have time to react. Somehow, his arm was sucked out the window. He was fortunate that there was uneven ground. If he'd had the entire weight of the truck entirely on his arm, the damage would've been so much worse.

Several months later, he returned to the clinic, and the nurses took pictures of his arm. The hospital staff was amazed at the body's ability to recover and the significant trauma and damage received by Hector. Two weeks prior, he had been cleared to return to work. His arm was stiff with damage and scar tissue. It would never be as strong or stable as it had been before, but he was fortunate that his arm wasn't lost in an amputation.

The original report of a teenager stealing the dump truck was a different location and a different situation entirely. It had no bearing on what happened to Mr. Brosnan.

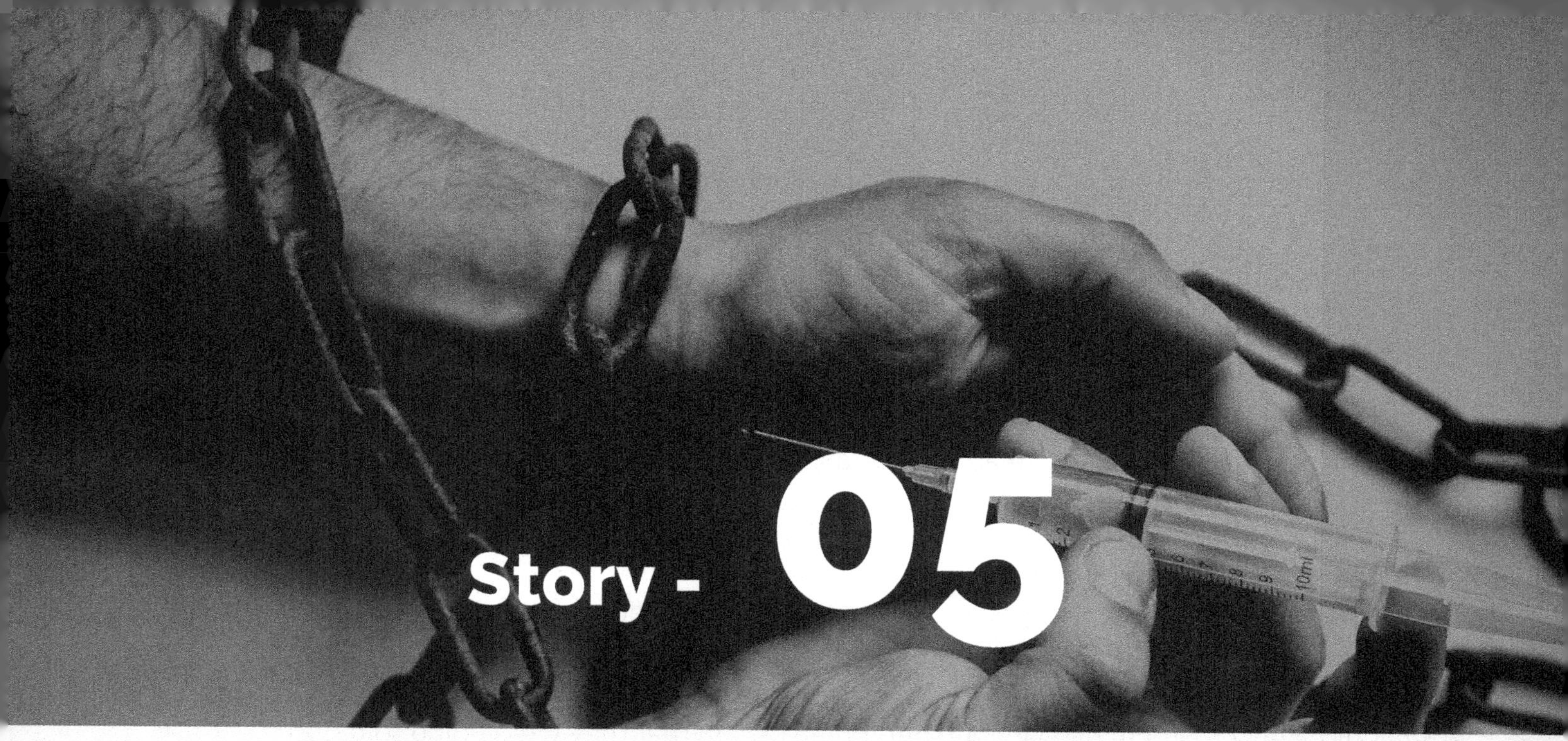

One Heck of a Lasso Swing

At a correctional facility near the ocean in a climate with heat and humidity, sometimes the inmates do spectacular things in order to attempt to change their situation or to manipulate their surroundings. For the staff, who have to work in these difficult circumstances, it can be tough.

A few years back, the nurses responded to an inmate refusing to cuff up at the door. They were there in case the situation became worse. The officers tried unsuccessfully for twenty minutes for the individual to cuff up. A social worker came who knew the inmate well, and within a few minutes, the inmate was cuffed and was brought out of his cell.

That was when the inmate, Zander Zenaway reported that he had swallowed fourteen small flexible pens, a portion of his razor, and two batteries that he had removed from the cordless phone, and more. Apparently, he had saved all these items and swallowed them within the last hour.

The nurses assessed Zander, and he was stable, but he reported some body aches, stomach aches, bloating, and spasms in his stomach. The nurses notified the on-call provider, and an X-ray was ordered. There wasn't X-ray capability on-site, and therefore an outside agency was called. It was a few hours before the X-ray tech arrived.

Once the X-ray was done, Nurse Elana spoke with the tech to better understand the situation. The X-ray tech reported that Inmate Zander wasn't lying. He had everything he had said and more stuck in his stomach. The pens might have been there even longer, but it didn't seem that they were going to pass.

A local hospital, almost two hours away from the prison, was called. A surgeon confirmed their fears, and the patient would require a procedure to go in, through the mouth, and remove the objects. If they couldn't remove anything, then surgery would be considered.

Zander was transported via ambulance to the hospital with an officer monitoring the situation. Zander was admitted, and it took a few hours before the doctor came to see him.

Doctor Rencart asked, "Mr. Zenaway, why did you swallow all these items?"

"I was hungry," Inmate Zenaway replied. "And, my section is so hot, there is no air-conditioning, and I haven't had food in two weeks."

Officer Davyan interjected, "None of that is true. He gets three meals a day, and yes, the prison is warm, but it's summer. There's air-conditioning in his housing area."

Inmate Zenaway responded, "Maybe, I just wanted a few minutes outside the walls."

Doctor Rencart and his nurses pushed Zander out of his room and towards surgery. Officer Davyan followed each step of the way.

Hours later, the retrieval of items had been completely successful. Surgery had not been required, but Zander was taking a few moments coming out of anesthesia. Doctor Rencart returned and performed an exam. Zander was considered stable enough to return to the prison. Quickly the transport vehicle and Officer Davyan sprung into action. Minutes later, with the help of the nurses, Zander was moved into a wheelchair and escorted to a correctional transport van, and driving back to the prison.

About thirty minutes from the prison, Zander said, “I think we need to pull over. I’m going to be sick.”

“What do you mean?” asked Officer Davyan.

“My stomach is on fire. I don’t feel very well.”

“From what?”

“I couldn’t help myself. I swallowed something.”

“We know. That’s why you went to the hospital. We already took care of that.”

“No,” Zander replied. “I swallowed something else after they removed the pens and stuff.”

“How’s that possible? You were cuffed the entire time.”

“I grabbed something when someone leaned over.”

“No way!” exclaimed Officer Davyan. “Is that even doable?” Unsure what to do, Officer Davyan called the prison, and it was recommended that he continue driving forward. Upon arrival at the prison, Zander was X-rayed again, and there was another foreign object in his stomach.

The hospital was called, and Doctor Rencart was far from pleased to hear that it was the same patient as before. Once again, Zander was transported back to the hospital.

This time, Doctor Rencart was far less conversational. He gathered the basic information of another foreign object but did not believe the story of Zander. He assumed that the patient had found something inside the van on the way back to the prison.

An hour after the procedure, Doctor Rencart returned to the room with a look on his face that was apologetic. He said, "Turns out that Zander here, swiped my nametag when I came in for an assessment. He swallowed the entire thing."

Officer Davyan replied, "When Zander isn't on his medications, he will swallow anything he can. It is impossible to stop him sometimes. It's not like the prison can remove all items permanently. It seems like the situation is only getting worse."

Doctor Rencart replied, "Unfortunately, this procedure was a little more difficult than the first one. He'll need to stay overnight."

"I will be relieved around midnight by another officer," replied Officer Davyan.

Zander loved the hospital dinner and asked for extra soda every twenty minutes until around eleven at night when Officer Davyan shut that down. He slept perfectly through the night without a single complaint.

Doctor Rencart returned early the following morning to discharge Zander. He asked, "How is everything?"

The new officer, Officer Martinez, replied, "Zander has been really anxious for the last hour. States he can't swallow."

"What seems to be going on?" asked Doctor Rencart.

Zander shook his head back and forth.

"Are you alright?"

Zander refused or couldn't say anything.

Doctor Rencart noticed that spit was coming out of his mouth and that Zander didn't seem to want to close his mouth. Performing an assessment, he found nothing inside his mouth, but it was clear that Zander was having trouble swallowing. A portable X-ray was immediately brought into the room, and Doctor Rencart was once again shocked at the image before him.

For the third time, in less than twenty-four hours, Zander had required a procedure to remove a foreign object. This time, surgery was essential.

It turned out that sometime during the night, and despite the fact that he was handcuffed, Zander managed to pull up his sheet and created a loop in his sheet. He swung the lasso several times from his hospital bed while the officer was either in the bathroom or during the change out. Zander explained that it took several times to lasso the blood pressure machine.

Zander yanked the machine closer and was able to reach a stethoscope. For over an hour, he bent a portion of the earpiece of the stethoscope and finally broke it. The piece was longer than six inches. He swallowed it early that morning. The problem was that it became lodged near the opening of the stomach and even cut into the wall.

Retrieval was not an option. Zander had a complete surgery where they were required to open up his chest and stomach in order to remove the entire piece dislodged in his esophagus and stomach. The surgery was complicated and required a full two weeks of recovery in the hospital and several weeks of only eating liquids.

Zander was moved to a particular room, with almost no extra items for him to swallow. Two and three officers watched him the entire time.

The prison only hopes that Zander Zenaway has learned his lesson and stops swallowing these foreign objects. Only time will tell.

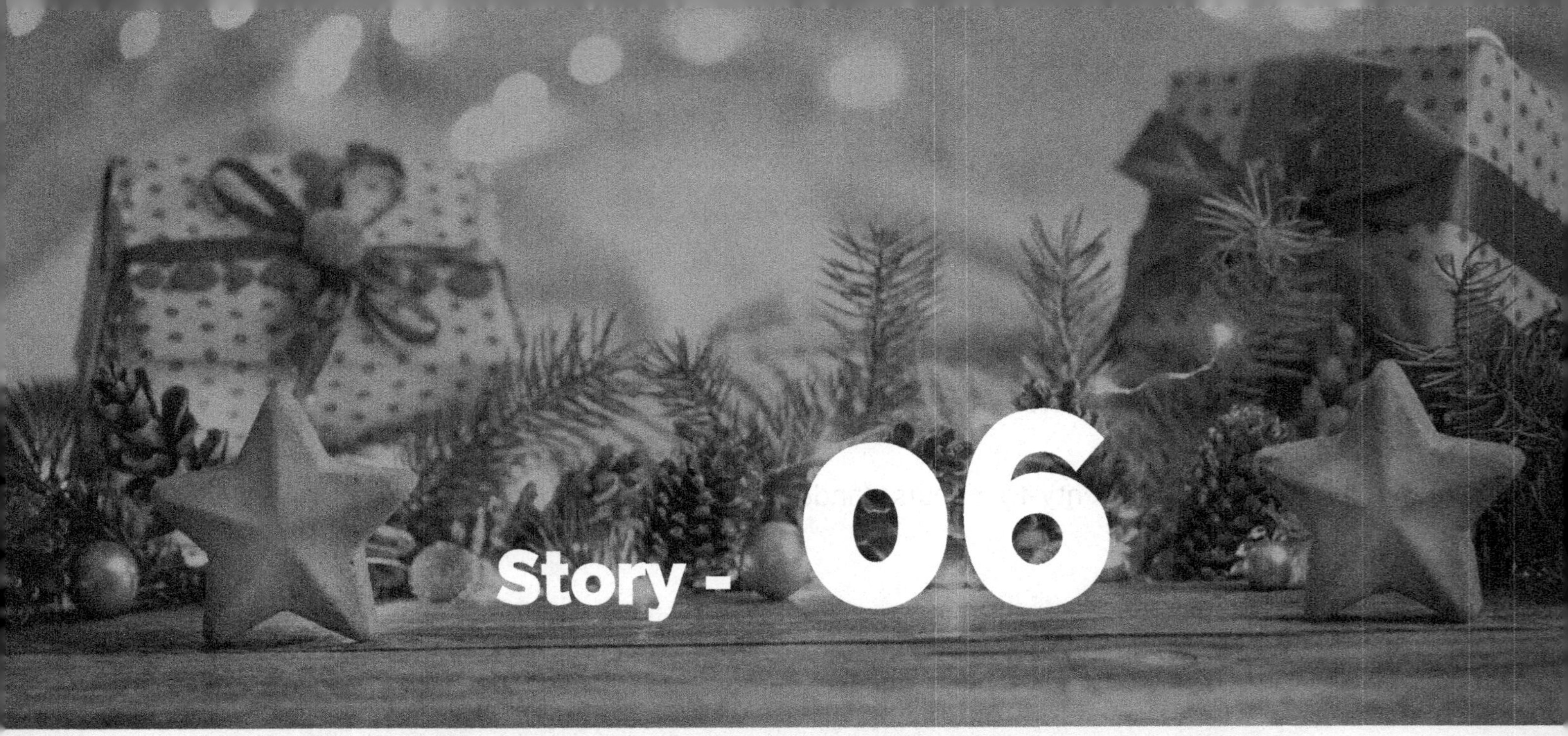

A Little Adventure When the Family Returns Home for Christmas

Grant and Dorothy were in excellent health for the most part. Over the last five years, they had relatively few medical problems or concerns. They had received their checkups and had done all the necessary preventative care requirements.

The most glaring thing in their life was that three months previously, their life had changed significantly. Their youngest son had left home to go off to college. That meant that they were now empty nesters. Two of their oldest children had been married in the last three years. They had two grandchildren, with a third on the way.

When Doug left for college, they felt a hole in their life for the first few weeks. They weren't sure what to do and how to feel about things. Slowly they began searching and trying new hobbies. They started to go to Applebee's every Monday night. They picked up pickleball and got together with their friends more frequently. It took a few months, but they were beginning to feel a little less lonely.

Christmas break arrived, and they were looking forward to having everyone back in their home. The bustling of crying babies and feet pounding up the stairs was a good thing. They knew that in another few days, it would all come to an end far too quickly.

One early afternoon, the day before Christmas, Dorothy came downstairs and began reporting to Grant that she was feeling off and short of breath. That rapidly turned to feelings of dizziness, feeling tingly, and having a dry mouth. At first, Grant thought she was having an anxiety attack about Christmas the next day or that she had overexerted herself cleaning and getting ready for the traditional Christmas Eve feast. But soon, Dorothy was lying on the couch, unable to keep her eyes open and feeling terrible.

Grant realized that this was an emergency. He called an ambulance, and it arrived a few minutes later. An IV was started, and Dorothy was placed on oxygen. This helped a little, but she was becoming increasingly difficult to arouse. Grant went with Dorothy in the ambulance. Only a portion of the rest of the family was at home. They would follow to the hospital a short time later.

The ambulance arrived at the hospital, and there had been no change to Dorothy. She was wheeled into the emergency room and a single cell room. The doctor came in and asked a few basic questions. Dorothy tried to answer the questions, but she was slurring her speech and was distant. It was impossible for the doctor to understand what she was saying. Her vitals were normal, and she was stable. The doctor turned to Grant and began asking about her medical history and what exactly had happened today.

Grant answered each question, and he could tell that the doctor was becoming increasingly alarmed. Because of her condition and her age, the doctor began a series of tests. The next hour or two was full of different tests checking the brain, heart, and plenty of blood work. She was given only a slight amount of IV fluids.

The family arrived and waited in the waiting room. Every thirty minutes, Grant would head out and give an update on which test they were running and the result of a previous one. About an hour and a half after Dorothy first arrived, Doug arrived. The family quickly caught him up on what was happening. Twenty minutes later Grant came out to give another update.

Grant said, "Good news, Mom is doing much better. She is still having trouble focusing, but she is doing good."

The family began cheering and hugging each other.

Grant continued, "Even better news. The CT showed that there wasn't a stroke. Nothing else is wrong with the brain. We are just waiting on some additional tests. Mom is still pretty dizzy, but she is able to answer most questions and is doing a ton better."

There were hugs and more cheers.

Grant turned to walk back into the emergency room when Doug came up to him. Doug said, "Hey, Dad. Can we talk?"

"Glad you made it. I have to get back in there to be with your mom."

"I really need to talk with you for a few minutes. It's important," Doug insisted.

Grant nodded.

Doug said, "Can we talk in the other room?"

"I guess. Is everything alright?" For the first time, Grant noticed that his son was looking sick. He was pale and sweating and appeared uncomfortable. "Are you feeling alright?"

"Oh yes, It's just that . . ." Doug shuddered for a moment and then went quiet.

"What's going on?"

"It's about mom."

Grant thought he knew what this was about. "Mom's fine. It was a little scary there for a minute. Blood work shows no heart attack. CT shows no stroke. They will watch her tonight..."

"It's all my fault."

"What are you talking about?"

Doug took a deep breath. "Earlier today, I think that mom was cleaning my room."

"I can imagine that she was."

"I had some candy in my room. And several pieces are missing."

Confused, Grant said, "What does that have anything to do with what is going on with your mom?"

"The candy isn't your normal candy."

"What are you getting at?"

"If you take a few of the gummies, it causes you to feel really relaxed. Can you ask mom if she ate any of these?"

"Are you saying that these are special candies?"

"Just ask her," Doug said, and he quickly walked away.

Returning to Dorothy's room, Grant didn't even have to ask. The answer was obvious as Dorothy was midway through the motion of putting what appeared to be a gummy worm into her mouth. Grant rushed over and prevented her from eating the candy.

The doctor was called into the room, and the situation was explained. He seemed to understand quite quickly what had happened. The moment Grant had said, "gummy," the doctor was nodding.

Dorothy remained in the hospital until early Christmas afternoon. With IV fluids, some medications, and a good night's sleep, she was feeling much better as she returned home. Doug was mortified, and he apologized profusely to both his parents. Later that night, after dinner, Grant whispered to Doug, "You don't know how lucky you were that the police weren't called."

"I've totally learned my lesson," Doug said. "Never again."

When the family went off on their separate ways a few days later, Grant and Dorothy were more than happy to see them go. They had earned a few months of quiet and relaxation.

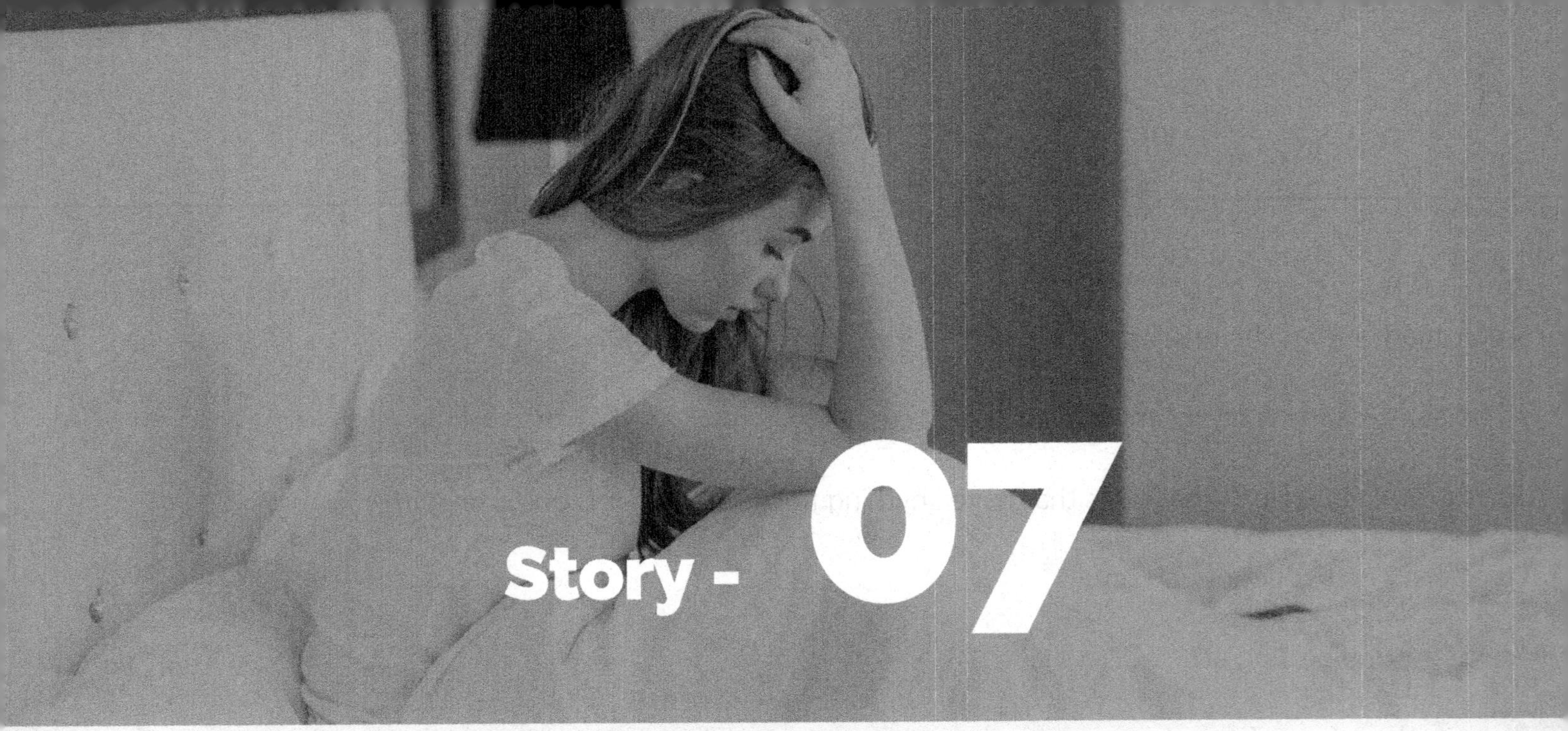

Story - 07

The Worst Headache of My Life

Doctor Welker stepped into the clinic's exam room and was surprised to see a former coworker's wife sitting in a chair next to the exam table. He did a double check on the name on the chart. He had been expecting to see George, a former administrator, though he hadn't seen him in ten years.

He walked forward to where the woman was seating, and asked, "Susie, how are you?"

"Oh. Hello, Dr. Welker. So good to see you. I wasn't sure if you were still working here."

"I'm hoping to retire in the next few years."

"That sounds wonderful," she said, full of emotion. "Congratulations!"

"Thank you. How are George and the kids?"

Susie replied, "They're doing really well. George has been so busy the last few months it seems like I barely see him. The kids are growing up so fast."

Looking around, Dr. Welker asked, "Is George here today?"

"No. He couldn't make it. He got called into work, but I came in his place."

"All right. Why don't I take you back to one of the rooms in the back? Would that be okay?"

"Sure." Susie was taken to an exam room. A nurse began getting her blood pressure as Dr. Welker said, "I hope everything is going well."

"Pretty well. I just started having these headaches the last few months that are life changing. When they happen, they are the worst headaches I've ever had."

"What kind of headaches?" he asked as he sat at his computer.

"It starts after I haven't slept very well or am feeling stressed. I get this weird vision in my left eye. Twenty or thirty minutes later, I feel the headache come on, pretty strong. Sometimes I throw up, and sometimes I don't."

"Have you ever been told that you have migraines?"

"I think we've all had migraines," Susie replied. "But these seem worse. I can barely get out of bed when they happen."

"Have you tried any medications, caffeine, or sleep?"

"Aleve and Tylenol. I think I even tried Excedrin Migraine."

"Did they work?"

"A few times. Honestly, I had to get some sleep, and that helped."

"How often are you getting these headaches?"

"Once or twice a week?"

"Have you gone through menopause?"

"Not yet thankfully."

Dr. Welker stood and added, "Can I do a quick exam?"

"No problem."

Several minutes later, Doctor Welker said, "Have you been running a fever?"

"I get hot and cold quite often."

"Have you had any change in your energy?"

"I feel tired all the time, and my nose is bleeding almost daily, especially on the left side."

"When was the last time you saw a dentist? Any recent dental work?"

"Maybe six months ago. I don't feel like I have any dental pain."

Dr. Welker took a light and checked all her teeth. Afterward, he looked inside both nares. As he was performing the exam, he said, "There seems to be a lot of swelling on this side of the nose and lots of bleeding. Any trauma?"

"Not that I can think of."

"Is your nose tender?" He pushed hard on the nose, and Susie pulled back.

She said, "That hurts a lot."

"I think we are going to run some blood tests and get an X-ray. Let's see how your sinuses look. Headaches can be caused by several different things, including dental pain, infections, sinus infections, and more. Are you okay with this?"

"I guess."

Fifteen minutes later, a nurse came in and took some blood, and fifteen minutes after that, Suzie walked down the hall to get a facial/sinus X-ray.

After what seemed like an eternity, Dr. Welker returned to Susie's room. With him, was two paramedics. Dr. Welker said quickly, "Susie. I think that we found the cause of your headaches."

Peering around the room, she added, "This can't be good."

"When was the last time that you ate popcorn?"

"Maybe a month ago."

"Did you choke on any?"

Susie took a moment to think. She finally answered, "I think that I did. George had me laughing so hard. I think a few popcorn pieces went up my nose. It took like twenty minutes to calm down."

"I don't think that you got everything out."

"What?"

"The X-ray shows a kernel is lodged in your nose?"

"How would I not feel it?"

"Well, you are in fact, feeling it. It could be causing your headaches, fatigue, nosebleeds, and more. I think you now have an infection."

"Can you get it out?"

"Not me. There's too much swelling and pain to get it out with you awake."

"Do I have to go to the hospital? Is that why the paramedics are here?"

"You have a temp of 102.9, and you're looking a little pale. It's a good thing you came in today. I called an ENT doctor over at the hospital, and you'll go directly into surgery when you arrived."

Susie asked, "Could you really see the kernel on the X-ray."

Dr. Welker called his nurse, and she brought the X-ray film into the room. He held it up against the window and pointed at the small kernel dislodged inside the nose. He said, "It was pretty obvious to see."

"Thank you, Doctor. I feel so embarrassed. I've had a piece of popcorn in my nose this entire time and didn't know it. Oh my..."

Susie had emergency nasal surgery. The infection turned out to be rather severe. She has a portion of her nose that required debridement or removal of dead tissue. The infection went into some deep tissue. The kernel was removed, but she required a second surgery after she recovered, six months later, to correct the damage done by the infection.

After plastic surgery, she ended up looking the same as before. She fully recovered and has no problems breathing out her nose. Additionally, she doesn't have continued migraines or nasal bleeding. She feels as good as ever.

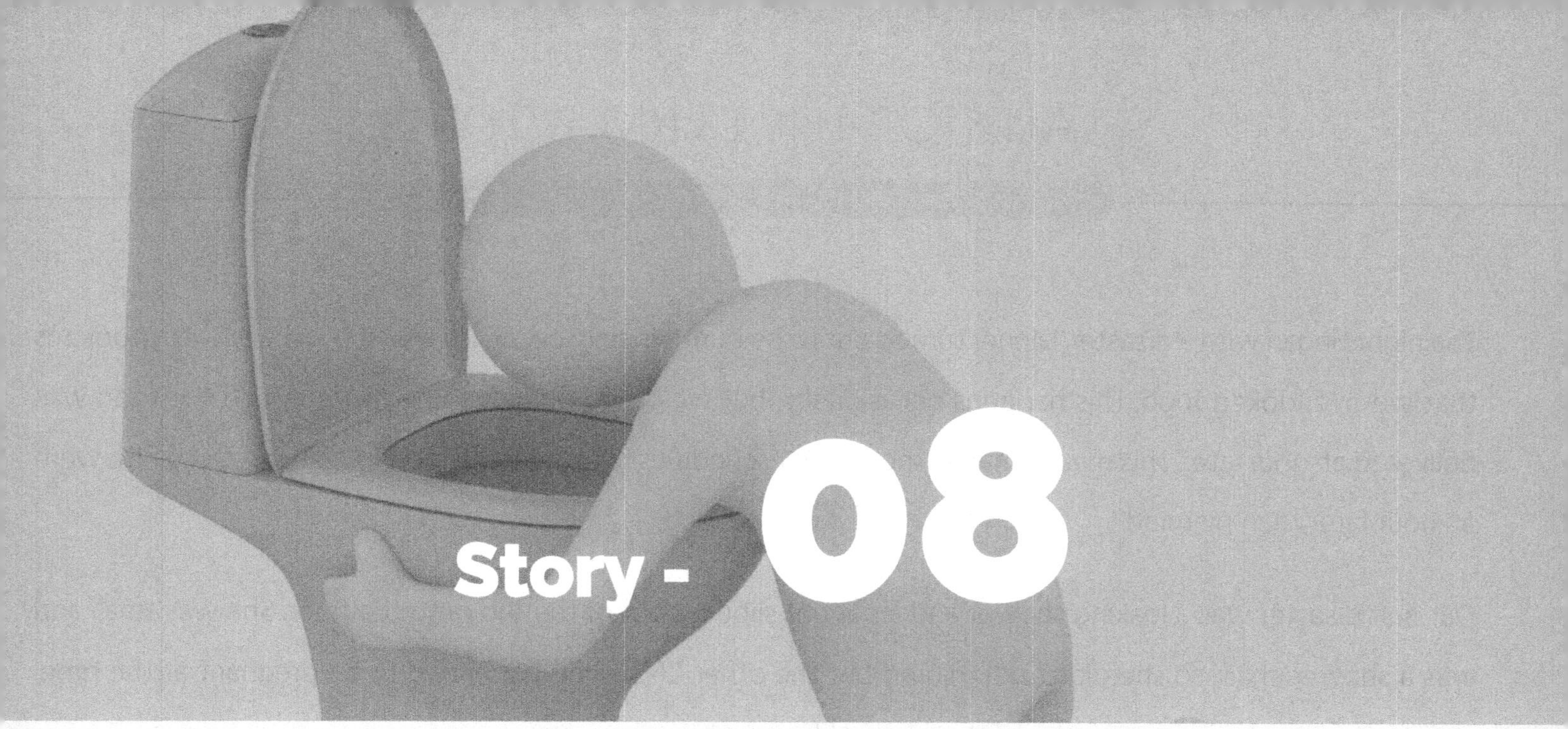

Story - 08

Vomiting Episode from Hell

Working graveyards in a nursing home are some of the most challenging work ever. It isn't a horror show every night, but often, one bad thing turns into fifteen. I've worked in several nursing homes, and each is different, and you have some unique problems, but there are some constants such as diarrhea, confusion, anger, vomiting, and lots of changing underwear and bedsheets.

You spend most of the night running from one emergency to another. There are nights when things are smooth and quiet, but that is a rarity.

Except for one night, there was a job that I absolutely loved because of my fantastic coworkers, it was a great facility, and it was really the only nursing home that was fully staffed. I worked there for years before I got into nursing school. However, the one night was one I will never forget. I was working with two of my closest friends, a CNA and a nurse. It was one of those crazy nights, going from one problem to the next.

The night began with a disaster. Dinner turned out to be burnt, mainly because we were so busy with problems that we overlooked food. This happens occasionally, but we called out for some takeout, and the food was delivered an hour later. This meant that all the shower schedules, walks, medications, and everything else were an hour later than planned.

Our first disaster was a leaking shower and a patient slipping out of the tub onto the floor. She was small and was a shower chair, so she didn't get injured but the other CNA, who happened to be pregnant at the time, got a fair amount of water on the bottom half of her scrubs.

The second incident involved a fight over which movie would be watched in our little rec room. Three men were fighting one lady over the movie. She wanted something different, but she also held the remote. The three men tried everything they could think of to get the remote from her, and she was accidentally knocked to the ground.

After that was settled, I was sent down the right hall to start showers and diaper changes for each room. This was the tricky part. I needed to stop at each room and shower those scheduled for a shower tonight and check the other patients to see if any required to be changed. The changing part happens three or four times during the night.

I was three doors from finishing when Becca, the pregnant CNA, called over her radio and said, "Sorry girls, it's time to meet outside Mr. Davenport's room. Hopefully, we can be done in less than thirty minutes."

Samantha, the nurse, and I had already agreed to help with Mr. Davenport. This resident had been sick over the last month and was on some heavy-duty medications. He was angry and spent most of his time in bed, watching television, or sleeping. It was nearing 11 pm, and we were hours behind our regular schedule.

The three of us met outside of Mr. Davenport's room after gathering our gloves, masks, trash bags, towels, and new bedsheets. We didn't think that things would turn out to be as bad as they were. Samantha had given him meds fifteen minutes earlier and had told him that we would come back for a shower, bed change, and new clothing. Mr. Davenport hadn't been willing to shower over the last week, but he agreed to the changes. Coming in as a group would give us the best opportunity to get things done quickly.

The moment the door opened, and we knew that we were in trouble. Mr. Davenport had been suffering from an intestinal disease, and something must've happened in the last fifteen minutes.

"I can't," Becca said, shaking her head. "What is that horrendous smell? Did he die?"

"Within the last fifteen minutes? Are you serious?" asked Samantha. "I'm sure that it isn't as bad as you think, and he is on your side."

Stepping into the room, it was clear that it was far worse than imaginable. He hadn't died, but it was the foulest possible finding otherwise.

Because of Mr. Davenport's bowel problems, he hadn't gone to the bathroom in several days. That all ended today and in an extra special way. This was the worst smelling diarrhea ever, and it was everywhere. It smelled worse than rotten eggs.

"Are you seeing what I'm seeing?" asked Becca.

"That much poo can't come out of one person at one time."

Covering my nose, I added, "The amount isn't the problem; it's the smell."

Becca was correct; she shouldn't have joined us. Less than a minute after seeing the diarrhea and smelling it, she was sent into a fit of vomiting. She wore a mask and couldn't react in time to pull it down off her face. She projectile vomited directly into her mask and all over her own face. Pulling down her mask, she began to heave onto the floor.

Samantha was the closest to Becca. "Oh no," she screamed, and it didn't take long for her to start vomiting as well. She must've lost her mind because she hustled over to the bed and started vomiting onto the sheets. Mr. Davenport didn't act like he was even awake or even knew what was happening.

I thought I had a strong stomach, but with two fellow workers and friends and the worst smelling diarrhea ever, I sprinted towards the bathroom and vomited everything I had into the bathtub. I first tried the toilet, but it turns out that Mr. Davenport had used the toilet and hadn't flushed. That made my stomach even sicker. There was no way I was sticking my head close to that.

Twenty minutes later, we had barely recovered. We had all eaten the same takeout and were now paying the price.

Becca asked, "Should we shower and change our clothes?"

"No," I said. "Look how much stuff we still have to clean. If we change now, we'll be changing again in an hour."

"This is the stupidest job I've ever had," Becca said. "Do they really think I want to clean up this mess?"

Samantha replied, "We don't get paid enough for this."

I agreed wholeheartedly with both of them. I asked, "Do we have those gowns we can wear?"

"Nope. This place isn't going to spend money on those things."

"After today . . . they better."

New masks and gloves were passed out, and we started cleaning up the room. As I said, when things go bad, they really go bad. Mr. Davenport refused to get out of bed for the next fifteen minutes and it took all our verbal judo skills to convince him to get out of bed. He weighed more than all of us girls combined.

I first cleaned the bathtub, but I was put in charge of the bed. Diarrhea and vomit were everywhere. I couldn't believe that I was stepping in and moving so much body waste. It took forever to clean up the room. I was close to vomiting another few times, and I think Becca actually did. She had the difficult task of getting off Mr. Davenport's clothing. She bagged everything that she could and threw away a few items. We immediately started a wash for his bedding and the rest of his clothes.

Hours later, the three of us sat together after each of us throwing away our scrubs and taking long showers. Luckily, I had an extra pair of scrubs because if I didn't, I probably would've quit on the spot. The only thing that got me through the cleaning process was the idea of a shower and fresh clothing.

Becca sat shellshocked and was the most traumatized of us all. Pregnancy had really affected her stomach, and we all agreed that we might have made it without incident if she hadn't thrown up first. We all cried at some point. Becca told us that she had sobbed and vomited at the same time when she was taking off Mr. Davenport's clothing. Turns out, he was super embarrassed and spent the entire time apologizing.

It was literally the worst day on the job I've ever had. We all got covered in vomit and diarrhea, and some of it was in my hair. Despite everything, I felt horrible for Becca. She went on maternity leave the next day and never returned to the nursing home. We are still friends and laugh at what happened, but it took a few years. We were all seriously traumatized that night.

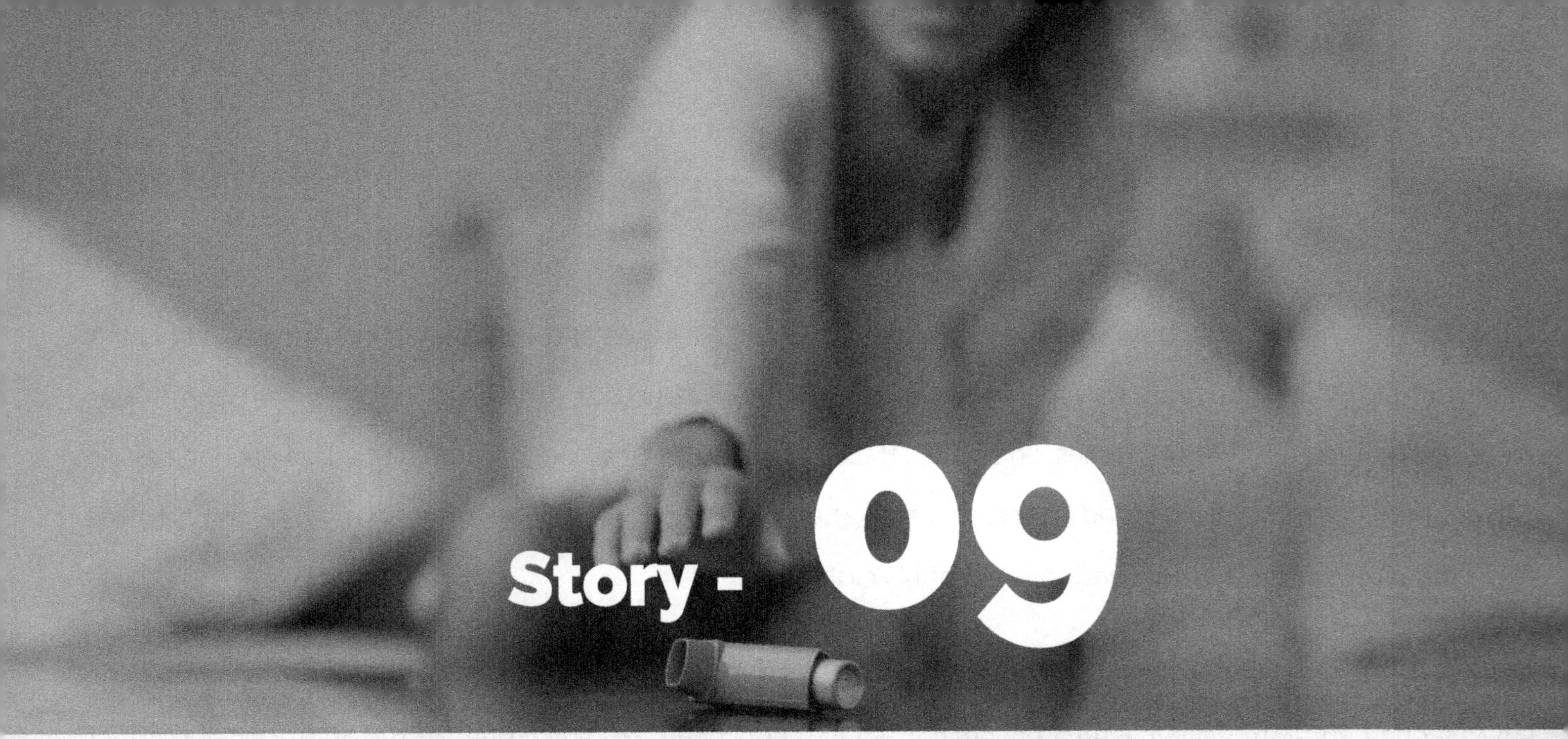

Story - 09

An Unexpected Cause of an Asthma Attack?

Brenda Jorgenson arrived at the local Urgent Care with shortness of breath and difficulty breathing. This was the third time this month that she had not been able to control her asthma through her inhalers alone. Her husband drove her to the clinic and waited in the car. He hated hospitals and hated to watch his wife struggle to breathe.

As she sat in the waiting room, she felt that things were getting worse. She got up and told the receptionist that she couldn't breathe, who immedicably notified a nurse, and the patient was brought back into a clinic room.

When they checked her oxygen saturation, it turned out that her sats (oxygen saturations) were in the upper 70s. The doctor was notified, and she was started on oxygen. After a quick explanation that she had asthma, Brenda received a breathing treatment called a nebulizer, to help reduce the inflammation and improve her breathing.

She remained in her exam room for the next twenty minutes, hoping that the breathing treatment would work and that she wouldn't have to be sent to the hospital. After the breathing treatment finished, her oxygen came up to 85%, but she was still wheezing rather noticeably. A second treatment was given.

Near the end of the treatment, Dr. Farley came in to watch the patient. Using his stethoscope, he listened to her breathing, both inspiration, and expiration. He noticed that the wheezing was not improving despite treatment.

He asked, "Have you been sick, Mrs. Jorgenson?"

Brenda shook her head.

"Is your asthma well controlled?"

Brenda shrugged, trying to imply—'not really, but I'm trying'.

"Are you a smoker?"

Brenda shook her head.

"I see," said Dr. Farley. "Let's get an X-ray and see if you have bronchitis or if it's just your asthma."

Twenty minutes later, she was pushed in a wheelchair into the X-ray room. She was moved into different positions, and a few minutes, she was finished.

By this time, the second treatment had finished, and Brenda felt her symptoms were worsening again.

The doctor returned to the room, removed an X-ray film from a sleeve, and put it up to a light. "What's this?" he asked, clearly concerned.

Brenda started to worry. She had a grandmother who died from lung cancer, but she grew up believing that if you didn't smoke, you had very little chance of getting cancer. She asked hesitantly, "Is it bad? Tell me it's not cancer."

Dr. Farley took out a second X-ray and put it up to the light. He said, "I don't see any cancer, but there is something that shouldn't be there."

"What do you mean?"

"Did you swallow anything on purpose?" he asked.

"No, I didn't." The question caught her off guard. "Are you saying there is something stuck in my throat?" Her heart rate quickened, and she started coughing.

Dr. Farley said, "Nurse Becky. Can you put Mrs. Jorgenson back on oxygen?"

"No problem, doctor."

Dr. Farley turned to Brenda and asked, "How long have these symptoms been going on?"

"I've always had problems with asthma, but the last month has been the worst."

"Before today, has anyone done an X-ray?"

Shaking her head, she replied, "No. I was given several breathing treatments and advised to use my inhaler more often."

He pulled up the X-ray to show Brenda, but she really had no idea what she was looking at. There were some dark areas and some white areas. Dr. Farley pointed to the left side of the X-ray and a noticeably circular object. "That looks like a penny."

"That penny is where, exactly? Are you saying it's inside my body?"

"It's sitting inside your lungs. Your right bronchus to be exact. If you see this area around the penny, I think it's causing you to have an infection. There's likely some inflammation and lung injury."

Startled, Brenda asked, "How in the world did a penny get into my lungs?"

"I've seen several pennies in children's stomachs and intestines. Often it is from swallowing them."

"I certainly didn't do that," replied Brenda, slightly defensive.

"I've heard of a case where an earring was accidentally breathed in by an asthmatic patient. Maybe that's what happened here."

"That's absolutely crazy," she replied. "What am I supposed to do?"

"We will need to get you transported to the hospital. They have a tool that they can go into the lungs and can retrieve the penny."

"Will it hurt?"

"I'm not sure you will be awake for the procedure. It probably won't hurt that much in the end."

Brenda was seen that day in a pulmonology clinic—a specialty with lungs. She was sent to the procedure room and was given a sedative through a vein to help her relax. The procedure took just around forty-five minutes.

The penny was removed, and there had been some damage and bleeding. It was likely that the penny had been in there for nearly thirty days.

When she awoke, she found her husband sitting in the room, reading a magazine. The doctor stopped by a short time later and explained, "The procedure was a success, and the foreign object was removed. You had some tissue damage and bleeding, which was expected. We will watch you for another four hours, and I believe you will go home on oxygen for a few days and an antibiotic. You will be feeling better by the week's end."

To this day, Brenda has no idea how she somehow swallowed a penny. It was unfortunate it got caught in her lungs, but she was fortunate that the outcome was so favorable. She healed up, and her asthma improved dramatically.

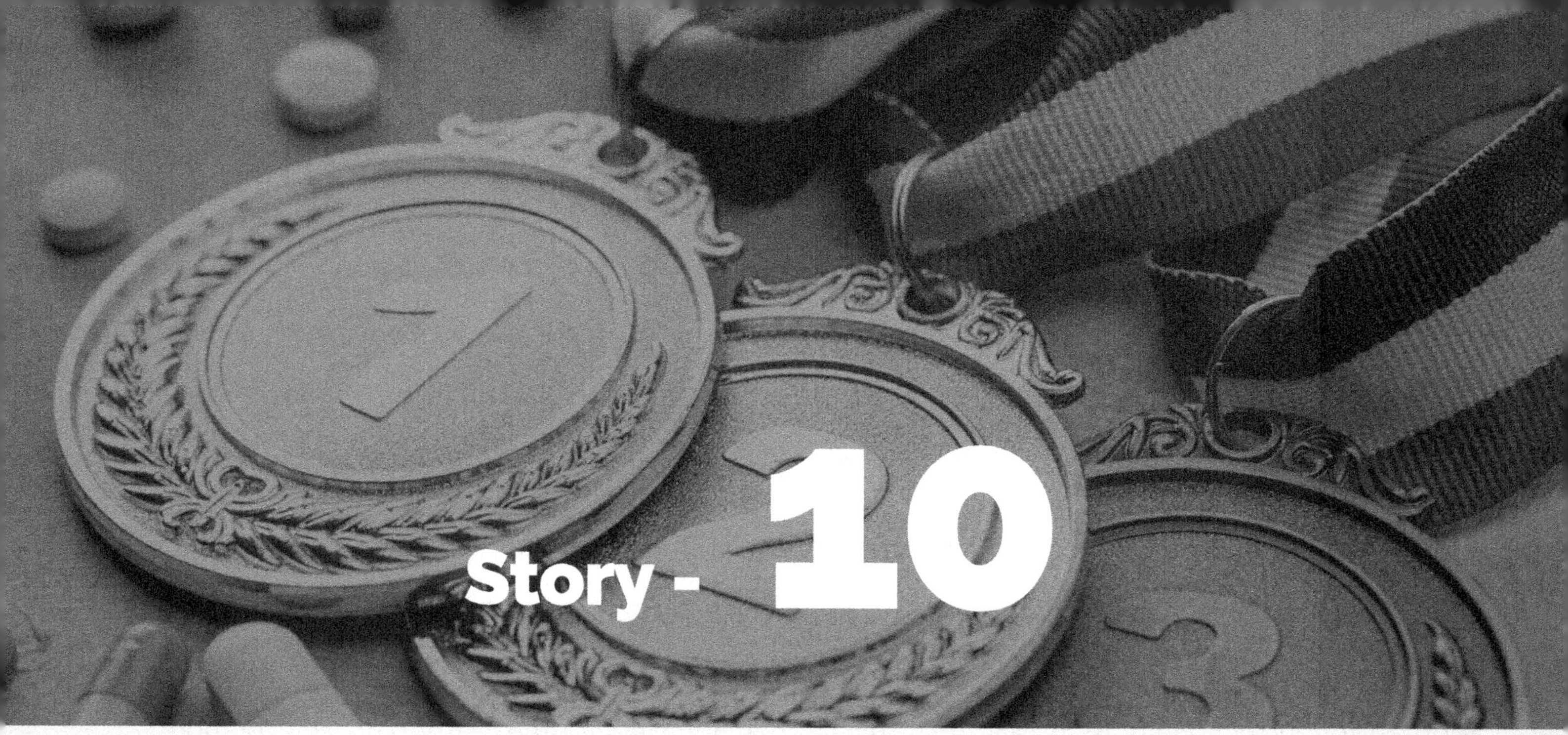

Story - 10

Gold Medal Winner for Ignoring a Problem

Inside the Emergency Room, we deal with many different problems and circumstances. Some of the patients that walk or are pushed through our doors had needed to see a doctor days, weeks, and months before they finally showed up on our doorstep.

This would be Simon in a nutshell.

Some background on Simon–he is homeless in Los Angeles and has been on the streets for years. He has schizophrenia and needs to take medications, but often he can't remember or doesn't want to take them. He has spent days at a time in different homeless shelters around the city but manages to find a way back to some of the places he likes near the beach.

Truthfully, the only reason why he came to the Emergency room today was that he was having trouble walking, and an officer noticed during a raid of a suspect that was believed to be hiding in the homeless shelter that Simon was at. The officer didn't find who he was looking for but found Simon dragging his right foot behind him as he crossed the street. The officer approached Simon and tried to calm him down. Simon didn't want to go to jail and didn't want to stop and talk to anyone. The officer offered to buy Simon something from McDonald's, and Simon, hesitating at first, finally relented and allowed the officer to buy him some food.

Simon and the officer talked about the Dodgers, the ocean, and their families. Simon's wife and kids had left him years ago after he lost his job because he could concentrate and finish the tasks that were being asked of him. During the custody battle, he wasn't allowed to see children, and after things were settled, he left the Midwest for better conditions in California. He had been homeless for the last two decades or more.

Officer Blackmon asked about Simon's foot, and Simon wouldn't say much but he admitted that it stopped working about a year and a half ago. He hadn't looked at it during that time, and if he ever showered, he didn't take off his shoes. Mostly he would walk into the ocean or spray something onto his head. The odor of Simon was strong, and it was clear that he wasn't healthy.

For Simon's sake, the officer handcuffed him and placed him into his patrol car. He assured Simon that he wasn't arresting him but was bringing him to the hospital for a wellness check. Simon explained that he didn't need to go to the hospital, but he didn't resist.

The officer called ahead and explained the situation. A wheelchair and a nurse were waiting for him when the patrol car arrived. Simon was brought into the hospital and taken immediately to an exam room. Once inside the hospital, the awful smell became more intense.

Dr. Fredrick and Nurse Lee were both sent to Simon's room moments after he arrived. Officer Blackmon remained behind if things became aggressive. There was no reason to arrest Simon, but they needed him to get the treatment he needed. Simon seemed nice and calm, but that could change in an instant. He was given some food, and that helped defuse the situation.

Nurse Lee asked, "Simon, how are you feeling?"

"Better today than yesterday."

"Have you felt sick in the last six months?" she asked.

"One day seems just like the next," answered Simon.

Dr. Fredrick asked, "Have you ever had surgery? Do you take any medications? When was the last time you saw a doctor?"

After these questions were answered, Nurse Lee asked, "What brings you into the hospital today?"

"Ask him," said Simon, pointing at Officer Blackmon.

"He can't walk. He's dragging his right foot. He can't place any weight on it."

"It's fine," interrupted Simon. "It doesn't cause me any problems. If that's it, could I get a ride back to the beach?"

Dr. Fredrick asked, "Simon, have you ever injured your foot? Spider bite? Or something else?"

"Nothing. I swear. It has never worked right from when I was little."

"Did you have this problem when you were born?"

"Maybe." Simon folded his arms. "Can't remember that far back."

Officer Blackmon asked, "Simon. What position in football did you play in baseball back in high school?"

"Shortstop and outfield."

"Were you a good hitter?" asked the officer.

"I hit second best on my team. I almost got a scholarship."

Nurse Lee said, "Sounds like you were really good. Do you like the Dodgers or the Angeles?"

"Dodgers. They are going to win the world series one day."

Dr. Fredrick replied, "We can hope."

Moving close to the exam table, the doctor tried pulling up the man's pant leg. Simon was unwilling to allow any type of exam. He pulled away, pushed, and lashed out.

"Can we look at your foot?" asked Nurse Lee.

"No reason to do so," Simon responded. "It is the way it is, and we can't go changing it. I'm done here. It's time to go."

Nothing that any one of them said made any difference. Simon did not want his shoe removed, in fact, he was adamant about it. They offered him a drink, candy, and much more. It was clear that he was going to resist anything they tried doing.

Finally, Dr. Fredrick left the room and called the hospital administration. He had only seen a small portion of the leg, but he was extremely concerned about the color of the skin. Fifteen minutes later, he was approved to give a sedating shot to Simon. Returning ten minutes later with two other security personnel and two nurses held Simon down and gave him a shot.

Simon screamed, "You're killing me. You're killing me. I'm dying."

When Simon was finally sedated enough, the staff began removing his shirt and such. They were unable to remove his pants or socks. Even the removal of his shoes was difficult. They began cutting off clothes, mainly his pants and his socks. Simon smelled awful; a combination of sewer, urine, and decay.

Simon had scars on his back and arms, likely from tree branches and fences. He had a left arm that was deformed, likely, he had previously broken his arm and didn't get the treatment that he needed. He has sores on his buttocks, groin, and upper thighs.

But when they removed his right socks, the medical staff and security staff viewed something they had never seen before. In fact, they weren't sure how it was even possible. Simon had a badly injured ankle and foot. The skin of the ankle was tightly attached to the bone. Most of the muscle and fat was gone, and the skin below the ankle was completely gone. All five of his toes had large portions of the bone that were exposed. The bone was discolored. Near the foot portion, there was some dry cartilage and ligaments that had fused to the bone.

"How is these even possible?" asked Dr. Fredrick. "I've heard about some drugs causing something like this, but I can't imagine how he survived this long." The doctor inspected the leg and found that blood flow in this area was largely diminished from the knee and below. The skin was cool but not cold. He was getting some blood flow to the leg but not to the foot. There were no bleeding or other signs of life in the foot itself. It looked like a cadaver's foot that is used in anatomy class or during Halloween.

"What are we going to do?" asked Nurse Lee.

"We need to get some blood samples, start an IV, and prep for surgery."

Simon required three surgeries, and most of his right leg was amputated. They started at below the knee, but over the next month, he needed two more surgeries. Simon was admitted to the hospital, and several lawyers, a judge, and a team of medical personal were assigned for his treatment. For the first few weeks, after the first surgery, he still refused care. However, it was felt that he needed the treatment, and a judge signed for the hospital to assume control over his decision-making.

Later, surgery was done to fix his arm, and a plate was placed. He was started on Anxiety, Depression, and Schizophrenia medications. Over time these helped, and the fuzziness of his mind cleared. He continued to have outbursts, anger, and paranoia episodes.

He relented and admitted that he'd stepped on a nail month and months ago. He got really sick but didn't want to go to the doctor. It would swell up and bleed. He would shoot up drugs into his foot and leg to help with the pain. At some point the foot stopped hurting, and he rarely looked at it or even thought about it. In the back of his mind, he knew that it was bad, but he decided he was going to die or it was going to stop hurting. When it stopped hurting, he stopped worrying about it.

Two months after he came to the hospital, Simon was released. He is still homeless, but he now has a wheelchair. He has long since stopped taking his medications. But officer Blackmon or some of the other officers will see him and buy him lunch every once in a while. Simon has been taken to a homeless shelter, and attempts to get him social security and disability have failed. Simon still doesn't want help and would prefer living on his own by the beach or somewhere else.

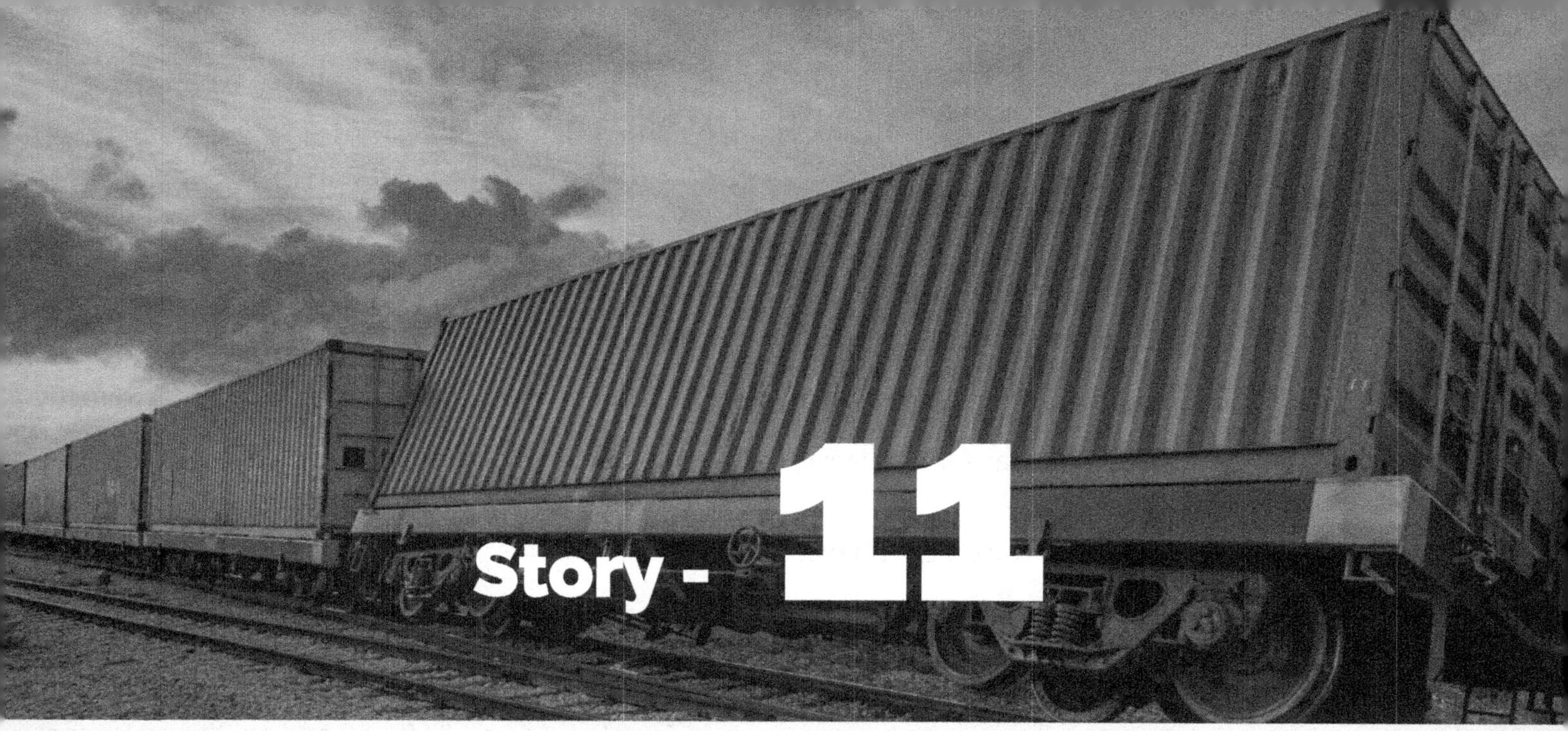

Story - 11

A Train Station Disaster

Every one of my worst days in medicine started as a typical day. Five years ago was no exception. The hospital I worked at was in the center of a busy city. There was almost no parking for the staff, especially those of us without the title of administrator. There was a mall close by and a train station. Honestly, parking and driving in this area were a mess.

I woke up at my standard time and took the city bus to work. It dropped me off directly in front of the hospital. Walking into the emergency room, I hoped that the day was going to go well. It never goes smooth as there is always something unpredictable that happens.

However, the things that happened that day were a level or two above unexpected.

I was assigned to help with three rooms in the emergency room. I was working hard with the doctor, a CNA, and we were seeing a lot of patients. I had started six IVs, sent three patients for various CTs, and had given out a lot of medications. None of my patients for the day had yet been required to be admitted to the hospital. That's always some extra paperwork.

Around 2 pm, just after I returned from lunch, everything changed. I was roaming the halls when a police car drove up to the front doors. Two officers jumped out, and one of them saw me right away and sprinted directly toward where I was standing. He was tall and lanky, but he was pale and bordered on hysterical.

He began screaming, "You've got to come with me."

"Where?" I asked.

The officer continued, "You need to get an emergency bag. Supplies, Gauze, IV fluids, and anything else that you can."

"What's wrong?" I asked.

"There's been a terrible accident."

"Do I need to go with you?"

"Yes. There's a pileup on the interstate, and the closest ambulance is twenty minutes away. I'm not sure we have that much time."

The officer wasn't able to say much more. The news spread quickly, and as I grabbed a ton of supplies, two other nurses were collected, and the three of us hurried to the patrol car. The doors didn't completely shut before we peeled out down the street.

The second officer, the one driving, provided a little more information. He said, "There's a drunk kid down by the train station. We think that he's stuck and badly injured."

The patrol car hurried down the street and turned right. Instead of going directly to the front doors of the train station, he turned left and headed away from the main building. There were other police already on scene, and they guided us over a utility road, across two train tracks, and directly to one of the main lines. Already, there were five or six trains parked on different tracks. None of these trains were occupied or in use, but they were there.

Approaching the sixth track, I noticed a fire truck had just arrived. A group of firefighters were being shown where to go. The patrol car parked, and we grabbed our stuff and followed. The group continued for about five or six cars along the track to where another group was positioned. A canopy had been set up. There were a few people, appearing panicked, unsure what to do.

I could see that they were pointing under the train car and explaining what had happened. My stomach dropped. When we were close enough, I heard what was being said.

"The kid is conscious. He must be twenty or twenty-one. He's been drinking, and I think he was trying to get back to campus. He says he lives on campus. Instead of going around the station, he cut across. The only way to cross was to crawl under the train. It shifted or started moving, and now he's stuck."

A firefighter asked, "How can we help?"

"You are going to need to get him out. He's stuck pretty bad."

"Where's the ambulance?" asked a female firefighter.

The officer in charge said, "Won't be here for fifteen minutes. We got some medical help from the hospital. They are right behind you."

All eyes turned to me and the other two nurses. We had had plenty of experience with emergency situations and the ability to just flow onto a scene and make quick decisions. None of us even stopped at the group. I yelled, "Where is he?"

Someone pointed to the area under the train where the young student was stuck. It wasn't a simple position. He had made it partway through and had gone past the first metal wheel, but that was when it had rolled onto his left leg, caught it, and had pulled the leg up into a space above the wheel. Blood was dripping onto the track. The boy was barely conscious and barely alive.

Jeff, a trauma nurse, said, "I'm going to come at him from up the track, and you go below." Turning to Zander, he said, "You'll need to stay outside the area and hand in any supplies."

"Done," Zander replied.

I pulled out a backpack of supplies and army crawled under the train. The boy's leg was mangled, but he had almost rolled onto himself. His head faces away from me. The only way he got in this position was if he also dislocated his hip.

The firefighters began working on the wheel itself. Their goal was to extricate him from the train. It was not going to be an easy thing.

"It's pretty tight in here," shouted Jeff. "I'm going to have a tough time getting him out."

"The only way he is coming out is if we cut off his leg or the firefighters find a way to move the train."

Jeff added, "He's losing a lot of blood."

I replied, "I don't have a good angle for the IV. I'm going to try to a tourniquet on his leg."

"I think I can get the IV, but it is so dark in here."

Yelling out to the other nurse, I said, "Zander. Get under here with a flashlight. We need to start an IV."

"Coming," Zander yelled back.

The boy asked, "Am I going to die?"

"How much pain are you in?" I asked as I pulled over my backpack and unzipped it.

"So much." The boy began crying.

I pulled out some IV supplies and passed them over to Jeff. We already had on gloves, but mine ripped as I crawled under the train. I pulled out more and put them on over my first pair of gloves.

To the boy, I said, "We are going to start working on you. We need to stop the bleeding. We'll start an IV and give you some meds."

"Hurry," the boy whimpered. "The pain is too much."

The tourniquet that I had in my bag was similar to a blood pressure cuff with a cord or wrap to pull tight. I scooted up to the leg, which was shredded. The jeans the boy wore were destroyed and soaked with blood. Bone was sticking out in a bunch of different directions. Blood was dripping everywhere. I unwrapped the tourniquet, and it took me a minute to find a place well above his knee to place it.

His lower leg bones below the knee were broken, and I was pretty sure his hip was dislocated. I wrapped the main portion around his thigh and pulled the strap tight. There was a noticeable change in blood flow, and it slowed significantly.

The boy screamed loudly and just about fell unconscious.

"This sucks," Jeff yelled.

Zander had come from a different direction and was pointing a flashlight at the boy's left arm. It was slightly trapped under the boy's body, but the right arm couldn't be moved correctly to get a good look at the elbow area.

"I almost got it," Jeff replied.

Zander shouted, "You got it."

"Hook up the bag to the bottom of the train. We will need to roll the boy more onto his back."

"That's going to be hard," I said.

"We have to try."

I reached over and grabbed the boy's shoulder and rolled him a few inches. He screamed again, and the way his leg was caught, he couldn't go much further.

From outside, a firefighter yelled, "We can't find a way to extract the kid."

Things were getting dire. We tried everything we could to get the boy comfortable and stable. We gave him fluids, pain medications and began wrapping his leg. That turned out to be pointless. Luckily a doctor had overheard what had happened. He came with the appropriate equipment.

I ended up sliding out from under the train. The doctor went in and cut the leg, causing an amputation just below the knee. He tried preserving as much tissue and bone as possible.

The ambulance arrived just as we were pulling the boy out. He didn't look good and had lost consciousness at this point. He was placed on the gurney, and the doctor rode back to the hospital with the boy. He went into surgery pretty quickly.

In the end, the leg required further amputation, and it ended up being above the knee. He had broken his hip, causing the dislocation. He required surgery for this as well.

It was one of the most gruesome circumstances I've ever been a part of. I never imagined working on a patient in the field as the ambulance crew does. It was a peek into an entirely different world.

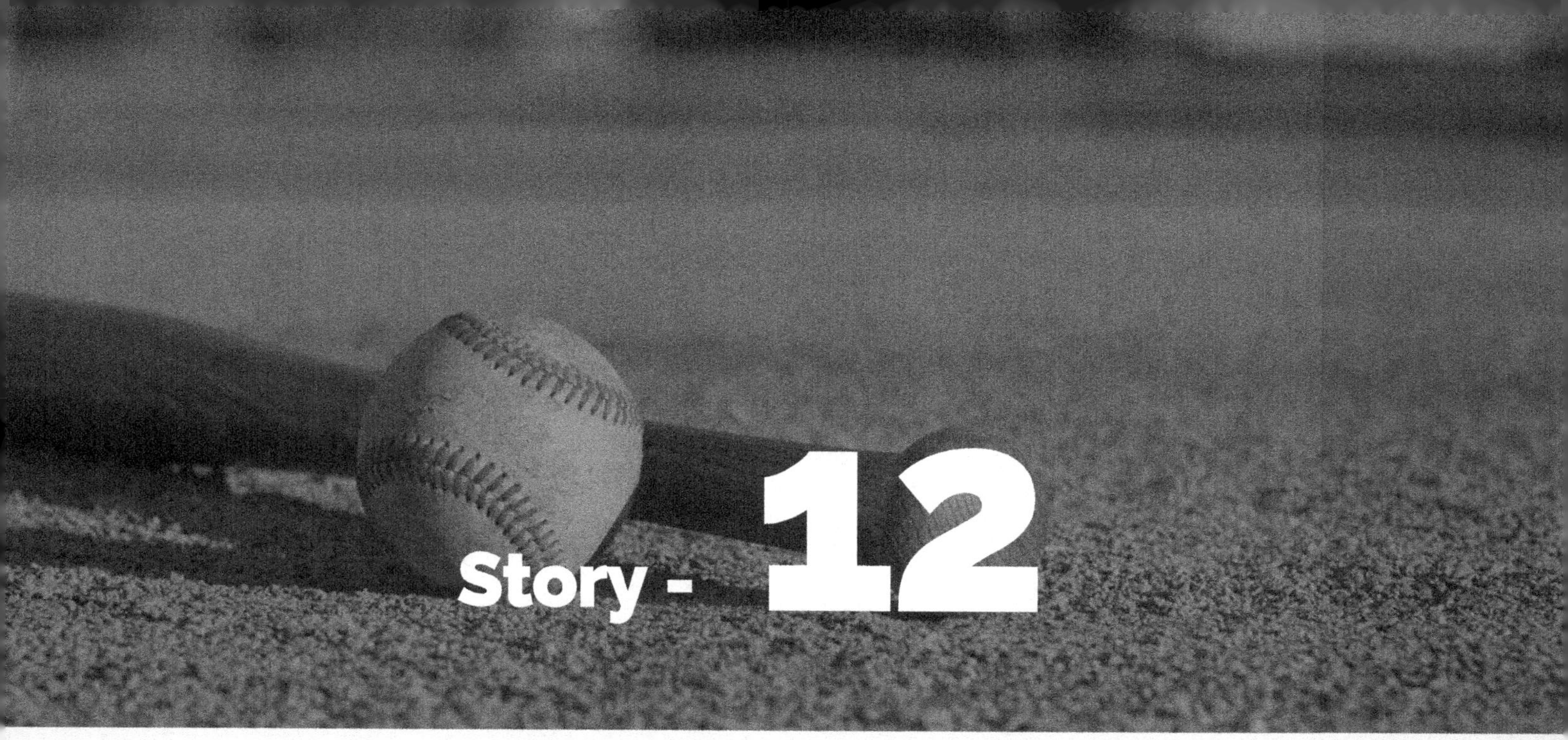

A Boy Playing Baseball Gets Hit in the Chest

Working in medicine and responding to a medical emergency on your day off is surreal. I work in Family Medicine, and one day I was at the ballpark watching my son play baseball. He is twelve and just started a few years earlier.

On a field next to mine is where the emergency situation took place. I didn't see it directly, but I was quickly told what had happened when I arrived at the scene. Any lack of action could have been disastrous to an already delicate situation. It was also surprising how many people did not know what was happening. It is vital that we all become more aware!

The player affected was the pitcher. His name is Dougie, and he was a good pitcher and a promising young man.

His game was in the fifth inning, and there was no one out and one person on first base. He had been doing a good job in the game. He had struck out three. The game was tied 4-4. He threw his pitch to the batter, who hit the ball directly back at the pitcher.

Dougie tried catching the ball and turned his body forward. I guess normally he would have been sideways with his left shoulder toward home plate. He tried catching the ball but missed, and the ball ended up hitting him directly in the chest.

This type of play has happened many times before. Whether in the field, pitching, catching, or even batting, a player gets hit with the ball in the chest. Most of the time, he or she gets up with a bruised chest and a bruised ego.

However, for Dougie, this did not happen. The ball thudded against his chest, probably the left side, but once he fell down, he did not get up again. In fact, his heart stopped working. There was a slight delay as most onlookers did not know what was happening. The players and coaches reacted first, followed by some of the fans.

That's when the screaming started. I heard the screaming from the other stands and sprinted around, trying to find out what was happening. I assumed a player had injured his ankle sliding into a base. I've heard that type of screaming before.

However, the crowd was near the pitcher's mound. I sprinted to the pitcher's mound, where the crowd had gathered.

Dougie was already turning a whitish blue. It was clear that he was not getting any air. I quickly felt for a pulse and listened for a heartbeat. Hearing and feeling nothing, I placed him on his back and started doing chest compressions.

Someone tried knocking my hands away, saying, "He was hit in the chest. You are going to make things worse. What happens if he has cracked ribs?"

Someone else added, "There are too many people around the boy. Just give him some room, and he'll be all right. The boy just needs to catch his breath."

"What happened?" I demanded.

One of the baseball coaches kneeling down explained, "The batter hit a ball that hit Dougie in the chest. He dropped to the ground immediately and stopped moving."

"Call an ambulance," I said. "I'm a doctor, and you need to call the ambulance right now."

The entire time, despite whoever tried pushing my hands away, I continued CPR. I gave him some breaths of oxygen, but only a few, and continued chest compressions.

Truthfully, my compressions likely did little to help Dougie, though I'd like to think that they helped. Luckily, an ambulance was really close by, and they arrived at the scene a minute after the phone call was placed.

"I'm a doctor," I said to the oncoming paramedic. "This boy took a baseball to the chest, and his heart isn't working. We need a defibrillator."

The paramedic agreed, and quickly the boy was placed on a backboard, and a defibrillator was used. The paramedics took over the care of the boy. As they continued working on the boy, he was moved to the back of the ambulance.

The use of the defibrillator is likely what saved the boy's life. Dougie was loaded up in the ambulance and taken to the local hospital. They wasted no time from the moment they arrived to when they left.

Dougie had what is called Commotio Cordis, a condition of impact at the heart at the precise moment – something like 15 milliseconds between beats can cause the heart to stop working. It has been talked about in medical circles for hundreds of years. They also did studies in the '30s. But it came more to the forefront back in the 1990s following a series of articles, but it wasn't until the internet that it became more commonly known.

However, by the reactions of the parents I was around, many are still unaware of this condition.

Often the impact is blunt and can happen from a ball, a bat, or something else. The condition causes the heart to go into an arrhythmia and stop. It was one of the scariest things I've seen.

This condition is often seen in those who play baseball and lacrosse but can happen in almost any sport. It doesn't have to happen in sports alone, and other cases have been seen in car accidents, child abuse, falling from a tree, and more.

Dougie was one of the lucky ones. Almost 70% of the individuals who get Commotio Cordis, the person dies. Around 15-20 cases happen every year. Coaches are being trained on the use of defibrillators.

Another important improvement is "heart guards" or "chest guards," and many children are starting to wear these protective layers over their hearts. They can be found online or at many sporting goods stores. Most look like compression shirts with plastic or extra padding. They can be lifesavers.

We all need to do whatever it takes to keep kids safe, especially if they are playing sports.

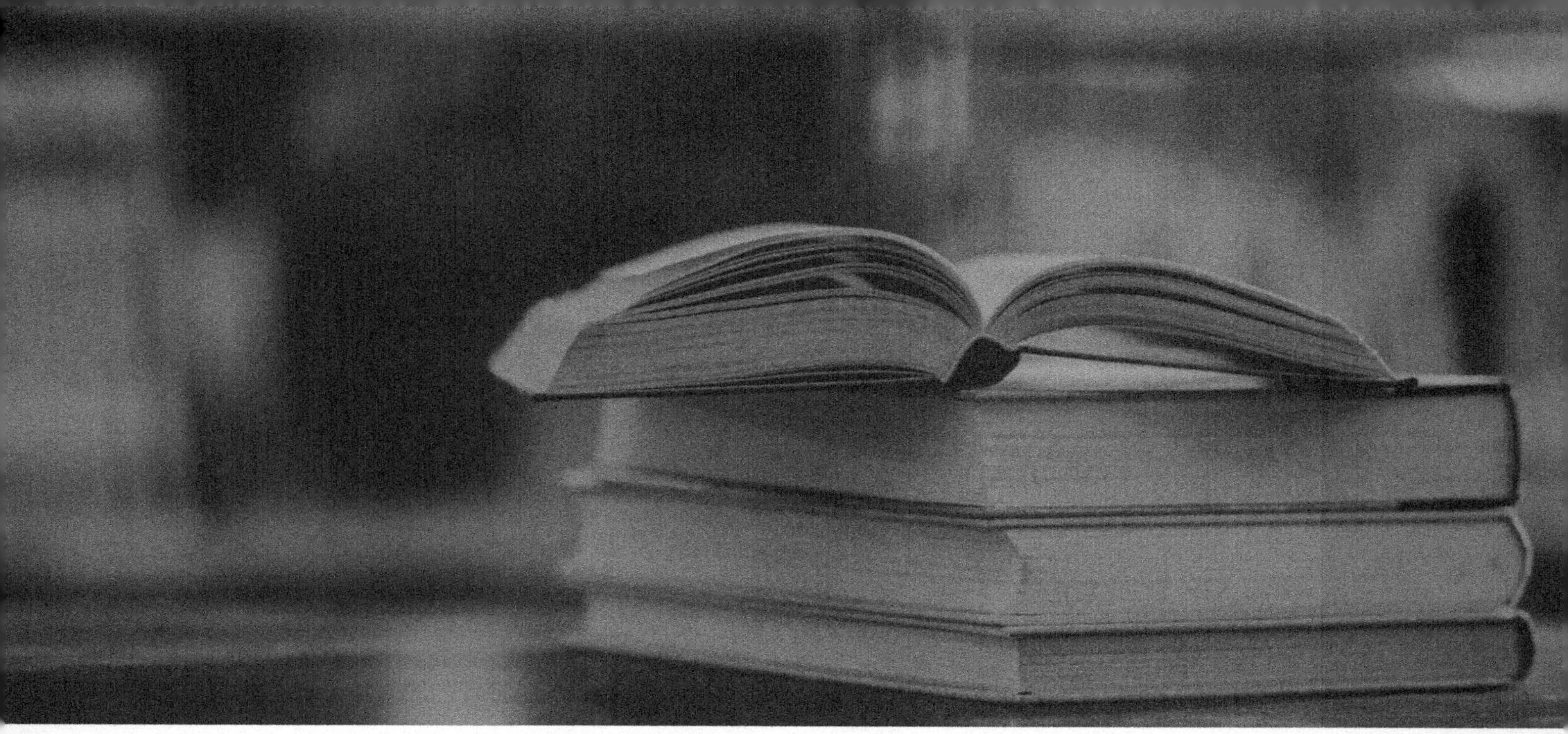

Tales of the Exam Room Collection

Check out our other Volumes:

***Crazy Medical Stories:* Tales of the Exam Room - Volume 1**

10 Short stories about the crazy world of Medicine. These stories have taken years to collect, understand, and write. Author Scott Kemp has worked tirelessly to bring for you this entertaining perspective of the patient and medical staff relationship. Each story brings about a greater clarity into the delicate choices presented day in and day out.

https://www.amazon.com/Crazy-Medical-Stories-Tales-Exam/dp/1736159844/ref=tmm_pap_swatch_0?_encoding=UTF8&qid=1618501286&sr=8-2

***Medical Horror Stories:* Tales of the Exam Room - Volume 2**

10 Short stories about the crazy world of Medicine. In Vol 2, we continue exploring the astonishing world of medicine as we discover some of the unpredictable situations between patients and medical professionals. Often, like a law of nature, when something can go wrong, it does. But the outcome is rarely as you expect it.

https://www.amazon.com/Medical-Horror-Stories-Tales-Exam/dp/1736159860/ref=sr_1_5?dchild=1&keywords=Tales+of+the+Exam+room&qid=1613685694&sr=8-5

***Medical Stories While Incarcerated:* Tales of the Exam Room - Volume 3**

12 Short stories about the crazy world of Medicine. Medicine happens in all shapes and forms. We are excited to present these stories centered around medical stories that happen in jails and prisons. But beware, these stories are a step or two more graphic than our previous stories. We have a long-standing love for medicine and some of the unimaginable situations that patients and medical professionals find themselves in.

https://www.amazon.com/Tales-Exam-Room-Medical-Incarcerated/dp/B08NYTQ6GX/ref=sr_1_4?dchild=1&keywords=Tales+of+the+Exam+Room&qid=1606499209&sr=8-4

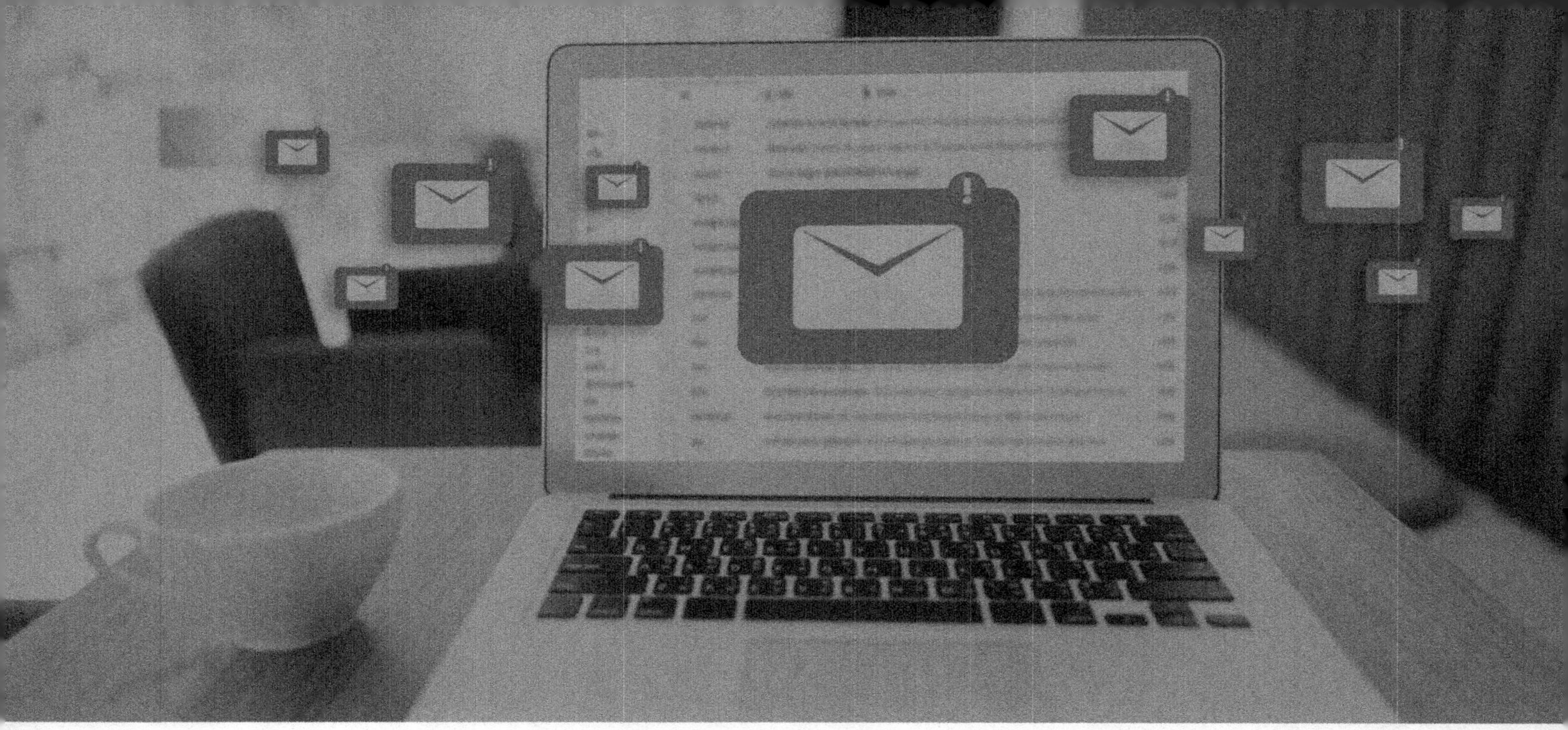

Sign up for our Newsletter

Join us at Exam Room Tales to get a better look at what we do. We will also offer special promos and you will receive benefits for signing up for our newsletter. Our team sends out a Newsletter several times a year.

The goal of the Newsletter is to keep our readers up to date on what we are working on. It also offers a platform to provide feedback, share stories, and much more. Our Newsletter team will also offer promos, special offers, incentives, unique stories, and more.

Come Join us at ExamRoomTales.com

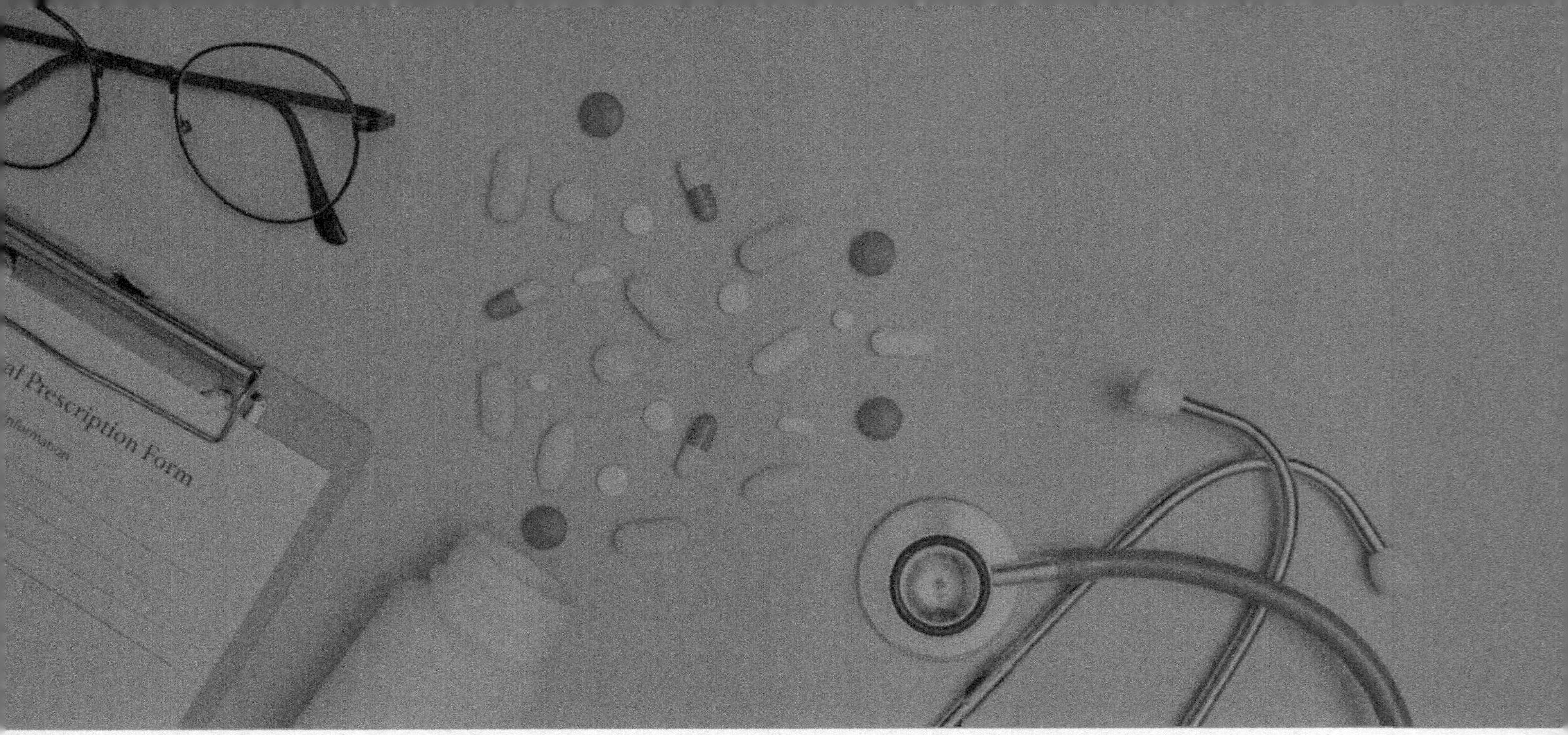

Correctional Medicine

The United States has, by far, one of the highest rates of incarcerations in the world. As of 2016 – 655 inmates per 100,000 are found within the jails and prisons of America. But other countries around the world are also experiencing an increase in the number of individuals incarcerated. Many different countries have tried different things to curb incarceration rates – some work, and some do not.

Each country has specific and unique ways to handle the medical needs required for inmates. This need may be overlooked or misunderstood when dealing with cost, workforce, funding, and many other areas of correctional responsibilities.

Additionally, millions of individuals have been freed from jails and prisons that are being monitored on probation or parole. This also adds to the responsibilities of the government, cities, towns, and communities. For those younger than 18 – there are often detention centers.

Correctional Medicine is challenging and unique. Inmates can be difficult to treat for several reasons, including risk factors, past medical histories, unique circumstances, unique mental health problems, difficulty following directions, homelessness, and many others. This isn't to say that every inmate falls into the category of being difficult. For some reason, the most unexpected things happen in prisons and jails.

Constitutionally, inmates should be provided with reasonable medical and mental health care. That means you can't lock them up and throw away the key. Many times, there are dental issues, pending surgeries, medications, serious medical and mental health conditions, and many more circumstances that should be considered and often continued if possible.

Not all medications that a patient takes on the streets will be allowed in a correctional facility. There are hundreds of different prisons and jails throughout the United States. This includes Federal prison/jails, state prisons, and many other forms of detention centers. Each facility will do things a little differently from one to another. This could be based on region, size, beliefs, medical knowledge, medical personnel, administration, financial, and many other things. In essence, what works for one jail may not work for another.

Medicine inside correctional facilities can be exciting, difficult, and even disturbing. It is rare when someone is satisfied with the level of care they are receiving, even if it is exceeding the standards available. Lawsuits are often brought against medical personnel, prisons, and jails. Some of these are for a good reason, but many are not.

The truth of the matter is that inmates are people and should be treated with appropriate medical care regardless of the crimes that brought them to the correctional facilities. On the opposite side of the coin, the medical staff is often attacked, berated, threatened, and more when they are trying to do the best job they can.

The following stories are intended to give the reader a picture into some of the crazier and unbelievable aspects of medicine. These stories are based on true situations, but many things have been changed to protect the patient. Some stories have been combined or changed to give the reader a better understanding and picture of the world of correction medicine.

To our knowledge, all patients involved received excellent health care.

Please enjoy!!

Made in the USA
Monee, IL
08 November 2026

67946270R00037